PHARMACOLOGY

for the

Boards and Wards

SECOND EDITION

PHARMACOLOGY

for the

Boards and Wards

SECOND EDITION

Carlos Ayala, MD
Adjunct Assistant Professor of Surgery
Uniformed Services University Health Sciences (USUHS)
Military Medical School
Chief, Dept. of Otolaryngology Head & Neck Surgery
MacDill AFB, FL

Brad Spellberg, MD
Assistant Professor of Medicine
Geffen School of Medicine at UCLA
Division of Infectious Diseases
Harbor-UCLA Medical Center
Torrance, CA

with Louis J. Ignarro, PhD
Jerome J. Belzer Distinguished Professor of Pharmacology
Nobel Laureate—Physiology or Medicine, 1998
UCLA School of Medicine
Los Angeles, CA

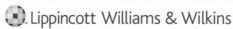 Lippincott Williams & Wilkins
a Wolters Kluwer business
Philadelphia · Baltimore · New York · London
Buenos Aires · Hong Kong · Sydney · Tokyo

Acquisitions Editor: Donna M. Balado
Managing Editor: Kathleen H. Scogna
Marketing Manager: Emilie Linkins
Production Editor: Jennifer D.W. Glazer
Designer: Holly McLaughlin
Compositor: Black Dot Group
Printer: R.R. Donnelley—Crawfordsville

351 West Camden Street
Baltimore, MD 21201

530 Walnut Street
Philadelphia, PA 19106

The publisher is not responsible (as a matter of product liability, negligence, or
otherwise) for any injury resulting from any material contained herein. This
publication contains information relating to general principles of medical care
that should not be construed as specific instructions for individual patients.
Manufacturers' product information and package inserts should be reviewed
for current information, including contraindications, dosages, and precautions.

Printed in the United States of America

First Edition, 2003, Blackwell Publishing Inc.

Library of Congress Cataloging-in-Publication Data

Ayala, Carlos, MD.
  Pharmacology for the boards and wards / Carlos Ayala, Brad Spellberg ; with
    Louis J. Ignarro.— 2nd ed.
    p. ; cm. — (Boards and wards series)
  Includes index.
  ISBN 13: 978-1-4051-0511-8
  ISBN 10: 1-4051-0511-9 (alk. paper)
  1. Pharmacology—Outlines, syllabi, etc. 2. Physicians—Licenses— United
States—Examinations—Study guides. [DNLM: 1. Pharmaceutical Preparations
Examination Questions. 2. Pharmaceutical Preparations—Outlines.—
3. Pharmacology—Examination Questions. 4. Pharmacology—Outlines. QV
18.2 A973p 2007] I. Spellberg, Brad. II. Ignarro, Louis J. III. Title. IV. Series.
RM301.14.A935 2007
615'.1—dc22

                                   2006007111

*The publishers have made every effort to trace the copyright holders for borrowed
material. If they have inadvertently overlooked any, they will be pleased to make
the necessary arrangements at the first opportunity.*

To purchase additional copies of this book, call our customer service depart-
ment at **(800) 638-3030** or fax orders to **(301) 223-2320**. International cus-
tomers should call **(301) 223-2300**.

Visit Lippincott Williams & Wilkins on the Internet: http://www.LWW.com. Lippincott Williams & Wilkins customer service representatives are available from 8:30
a.m. to 6:00 p.m., EST.

                                       07 08 09 10
                              3 4 5 6 7 8 9 10

We dedicate this book to Professor Louis Ignarro, a distinguished scientist, scholar, mentor, and true gentleman.

Preface

In medical school we were fortunate enough to study pharmacology at a time when Professor Louis Ignarro was the course coordinator and primary lecturer. Dr. Ignarro won the award for outstanding preclinical teacher at our medical school more than a dozen times before being granted the Nobel Prize in Medicine for his seminal research in nitric oxide biology. It is our privilege to work with him on this book, passing along his rich legacy of teaching to new generations of medical students.

In this book, we maintain our outline format to spare readers needless information and to save time for busy medical students and interns who need a quick, ready reference for review. No other book on the market so broadly addresses the needs of those taking the USMLE Steps 1–3 in such a concise manner.

We welcome any feedback you may have about *Pharmacology for the Boards and Wards*. Please feel free to contact the authors with your comments or suggestions.

> Boards and Wards
> c/o Lippincott Williams & Wilkins
> 351 W. Camden Street
> Baltimore, MD 21201

We hope you find this book useful on the Boards and Wards.

Contents

Tables

Figures

Abbreviations

$\rightarrow$	causes/leads to/analysis shows
$\uparrow$ / $\downarrow$	increases or high/decreases or low
1°/2°/3°	primary/secondary/tertiary
$\oplus$	positive/stimulates/turns on
bid	twice per day
Dx	diagnosis
DDx	differential diagnosis
dz(s)	disease(s)
hr(s)	hour(s)
HTN	hypertension
hx	history
IV	intravenous
mo(s)	month(s)
po	oral
pt(s)	patient(s)
Px	prognosis
qd	every day
Si/Sx	signs/symptoms
Tx	treatment
yr(s)	year(s)

1. BASIC CONCEPTS

I. Terminology

A. A drug = any agent administered to the body to mediate a biological response

B. A receptor = a molecule, typically a protein, to which a drug binds to mediate its effect

C. Efficacy = the maximal response induced by a drug—a more efficacious drug elicits a higher maximal response

D. Potency = the effective dose of a drug—a more potent drug elicits a response at lower concentrations than a less potent drug

E. Tachyphylaxis = tolerance or refractoriness to a previously effective drug that develops after prolonged use of the drug due to depletion of intracellular stores of the drug's target

F. Drug–drug interactions

   1. Two drugs are "additive" if the biological effect of giving both drugs at once is **equal to** the sum of the effects of giving each drug individually

   2. Two drugs are "synergistic" if the biological effect of giving both drugs at once is **greater than** the sum of the effects of each drug individually

   3. "Potentiation" is a special subset of synergy in which one of the drugs has no effect when given by itself, but when given in combination with a second drug causes the second drug to work more potently

   4. Two drugs are "antagonistic" when the effect of giving both drugs at once is **less than** the sum of the effects of giving them individually

G. Drug-receptor interactions (see Figure 1.1)

   1. Competitive antagonism

     (a) A competitive antagonist binds to a receptor without activating it

     (b) When a competitive antagonist is present, a higher concentration of agonist is required to achieve the same biological effect—**competitive antagonists reduce the potency of a drug**

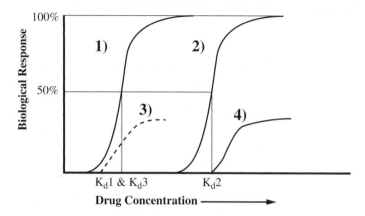

Figure 1.1 Receptor Agonism & Antagonism
1) A curve of biological effect vs. dose is depicted for a hypothetical drug, drug X. The K_d value for drug X (K_d1), which represents the concentration of X necessary to achieve 50% of the maximal response, is also shown. **2)** This curve represents the effect vs. concentration of drug X in the presence of a competitive inhibitor. Note that the maximum achievable response (e.g., the drug's efficacy, represented by the y-axis) is not altered by the competitive inhibitor. However, the drug's potency is markedly reduced, meaning that a much higher concentration of drug X is necessary in the presence of the inhibitor to achieve the same biological response as when the inhibitor is not present. Note also that the K_d is markedly shifted in the presence of the inhibitor; the higher K_d (K_d2) is reflective of a lower affinity of the drug for its receptor in the presence of the inhibitor. **3)** A partial agonist mimicking drug X binds to the same receptor with an identical K_d (K_d3), but despite its equivalent affinity for the receptor is unable to mediate the same biological response as drug X. The partial agonist has identical potency, but a much lower efficacy than drug X. **4)** Irreversible antagonism effectively reduces the number of receptors available for drug X, which causes a decrease in both the potency and efficacy of drug X and increases the K_d.

    (c) By definition, competitive antagonism can be completely overcome by increasing the concentration of the agonist— **competitive antagonists do NOT reduce the efficacy of a drug**

  2. Irreversible (noncompetitive) antagonism

    (a) Irreversible, or noncompetitive, antagonists bind to a receptor in such a way as to completely inactivate it

    (b) Irreversible antagonism decreases the maximum biological response achievable by an agonist

    (c) By definition, an irreversible antagonist cannot be completely overcome by increasing the agonist concentration— **irreversible antagonists DO reduce the efficacy of a drug**

3. Partial agonism
   (a) A partial agonist has the same affinity for a receptor
       as a full agonist, but has a lower maximum biological
       effect
   (b) Partial agonists bind to the receptor but have a weaker
       ability to induce a biological response
   (c) A partial agonist can also act as an antagonist (either com-
       petitive or noncompetitive depending on the nature of its
       receptor binding) to a full agonist

II. Pharmacokinetics

A. Pharmacokinetics is the distribution of drug in the body and its
   elimination by the body—**pharmacokinetics is what the body
   does to the drug**
B. Kinetics (see Figure 1.2)
   1. Zero Order elimination
      (a) Zero Order elimination occurs when **the rate of drug
          elimination is independent of drug concentration**, and a

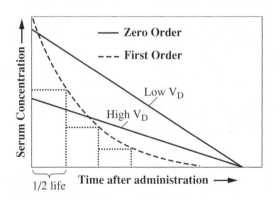

Figure 1.2 Pharmacokinetics
Zero Order elimination occurs when the rate of elimination of a drug is constant, having no relationship with the amount of drug present in the serum.
First Order elimination is achieved when the rate of elimination is proportional
to the amount of drug present in serum; at high serum concentrations the rate
of elimination is faster, and at low serum concentrations the rate is slower. First
Order elimination is quantified by a "half-life." Two lines representing Zero
Order kinetics are shown, one depicting a drug with a high volume of distribution (V_D), and the other depicting a drug with a low V_D. Drugs with low V_D
tend to remain inside the vasculature, so they have higher serum concentrations than drugs that diffuse out of the vasculature and into tissues.

constant absolute quantity of remaining drug is eliminated per unit time

(b) Zero Order elimination occurs without a constant half-life ($t_{1/2}$)

2. First Order elimination

(a) First Order elimination occurs when **the rate of drug elimination is dependent on the drug concentration**, with a constant fraction of the remaining drug eliminated per unit time

(b) The rate of elimination is faster when the drug concentration is higher

(c) **In First Order elimination the drug has a constant half-life**

(d) Elimination rate constant = $K_{elimination}$

(1) Only applicable in First Order elimination, where there is a half-life

(2) $K_{elimination} = \ln(2)/t_{1/2} = 0.69/t_{1/2}$

(3) Units of $K_{elimination} = time^{-1}$

(4) Example: for a drug with First Order kinetics and a $t_{1/2}$ of 4 hours:

$$K_{elimination} = 0.69/4 \text{ hours} = 0.1725 \text{ hour}^{-1},$$

which means that 17.25% of the drug is cleared from the serum per hour

3. Saturable elimination

(a) The body's ability to eliminate some drugs is saturable at commonly used doses

(b) These drugs can easily build up in the body on repeated doses, and dosing for these drugs must be adjusted based on the serum level of the drug

(c) Remember that the body's ability to eliminate a drug can vary depending on underlying illness—for example, in acute renal failure, the loss of glomerular filtration causes many drugs that are normally easily excreted to build up to potentially dangerous levels in the blood, unless doses are adjusted lower or given less frequently

C. Volume of distribution (V_D)

1. **V_D is a measurement of the tissue volume into which a drug penetrates**

2. V_D (mL) = dose of drug (mg)/concentration in serum (mg/mL) immediately after dosing

3. Thus, at a given dosage, **the V_D is inversely proportional to the concentration of the drug in the serum** (see Figure 1.2)

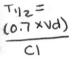

$$T_{1/2} = \frac{(0.7 \times Vd)}{Cl}$$

4. **Drugs that do not diffuse out of the vascular compartment have low V_D values, whereas those that diffuse widely into tissues have very high V_D values**

5. Lipophilic drugs, or those that do not significantly bind plasma proteins, have high V_D values

6. Hydrophilic drugs, or those that do significantly bind plasma proteins, have low V_D values

7. Because the average of volume of blood in a human is about 5 liters, a V_D of less than 5 liters indicates a drug does not leave the vascular compartment, whereas a V_D of greater than 5 liters indicates the drug does leave the vascular compartment

D. Clearance

1. **Clearance is the volume of plasma cleared of drug per unit time**—note the units of clearance are mL/min (milliliters of plasma cleared of drug per minute)

2. Clearance of a drug (mL/min) is equal to the drug's V_D (mL) $\times$ the drug's $K_{elimination}$ (min^{-1})

$$C \ (mL/min) = V_D \ (mL) \times K_{elimination} \ (min^{-1})$$

3. Thus, a drug with a long half-life and consequently a low $K_{elimination}$ is cleared more slowly than a drug with a short half-life

4. Conversely, a drug with a large V_D, which by definition exists mostly out of the vascular compartment, is easier to clear from the plasma than a drug that has a low V_D and thus exists mostly in the plasma—note that clearance of a drug from the body is NOT the same as clearance from plasma, because drugs with large volumes of distribution are easy to clear from plasma (because most of the drug isn't in the plasma anyway), but difficult to clear from the rest of the body

E. Dosing schedule

1. If repeated doses of a drug are administered, the serum concentration of the drug will build up in between doses until steady-state equilibrium is established with the drug's clearance (see Figure 1.3A)

   (a) When drugs are administered at a constant rate (either by constant IV infusion or by frequent oral dosing) the time to reach steady-state equilibrium concentration in the serum is directly proportional to the half-life of the drug

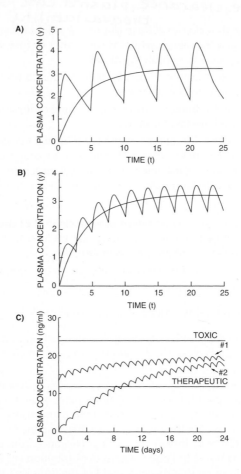

Figure 1.3 Steady-State Equilibrium & Loading Doses
A. As the doses of a drug are administered at a given periodic interval, the serum concentrations rise abruptly immediately postdose and then fall gradually as the drug is metabolized. If the dosing interval is shorter than the time necessary to metabolize the drug, the drug concentration will rise in the serum between doses, until a steady-state equilibrium is reached between the dosing interval and amount and the body's metabolism of the drug. This steady state is achieved quickly with drugs that have short half-lives, but more doses are required to attain steady state for drugs that have long half-lives. **B.** Identical average plasma concentrations are achieved with more moderate peak and trough levels when the dosing interval is decreased in proportion to a decrease in the dose. **C.** Because drugs that have long half-lives can take a long time to reach steady state with constant dosing, a shortcut is to give a high "loading dose" followed by smaller maintenance doses. This approach allows rapid attainment of therapeutic serum levels of a drug following one large dose, whereas dosing smaller amounts at fixed intervals requires much longer for the drug to reach therapeutic levels.

(b) **Thus, drugs with shorter half-lives achieve steady-state serum levels after fewer doses,** whereas drugs with longer half-lives require many more doses to achieve steady-state serum levels

2. **By halving the dose of the drug and doubling the frequency of administration, the same average plasma concentration is achieved at steady state, but the peak and trough changes following each dose are smaller** (see Figure 1.3B)

3. **To rapidly achieve a steady-state serum level of a drug with a long half-life, a large loading dose is given, followed by small maintenance doses** (see Figure 1.3C)

F. Dosing interval to maintain a steady-state drug concentration

1. For administration of a drug as a constant IV infusion, the dosing rate (mg/min) can be calculated from the desired serum drug level (mg/mL) × the drug's clearance (mL/min)

Infusion rate (mg/min) = desired serum drug level (mg/mL) × drug clearance (mL/min)

2. For administration of an oral drug, two new variables are introduced

(a) **Bioavailability is the fraction of administered drug that is actually absorbed into the body**

(b) The bioavailability of an IV dose is assumed to be 1 (or 100%) because these drugs are, by definition, completely absorbed, whereas oral doses may not be completely absorbed and so have bioavailabilities of less than 1 (<100%)

(c) The time interval between doses is also important for oral drugs (or for drugs given IV push at regular intervals, as opposed to drugs given by constant IV infusion, which have no intervals between dosing)

(d) Mathematically, the dosing frequency of an oral drug is calculated as the dose given (mg) × the bioavailability (a fraction <1.0, but lacking units), divided by the dosing interval (hours or minutes); this should equal the desired plasma concentration of the drug (mg/mL) × the plasma clearance of the drug (mL/min or hour)

Dose (mg) × bioavailability/dosing interval (hr) = desired drug level (mg/mL) × drug clearance (mL/hr)

Example: a 100 mg dose of a drug with a 75% oral bioavailability and a clearance of 1000 mL/hr should be given every 5 hours to maintain a drug level of 0.015 mg/mL

100 mg × 0.75/5 hrs = 0.015 mg/mL × 1000 mL/hr

(e) Thus, by starting with knowledge of the drug's bioavailability and its drug clearance, and knowing the desired target serum level, a clinician can determine the necessary oral dose and the interval of that dose needed to maintain the target serum level

G. Drug distribution

1. Partition coefficient

(a) Partition coefficient is determined by mixing a drug in a solution of lipid and water and calculating the fraction of drug contained in the lipid layer versus the aqueous layer

(b) Partition coefficient = drug concentration in lipid layer/ drug concentration in aqueous layer

(c) **Thus, drugs with high partition coefficients are more lipid soluble**

(d) Hydrophilic subgroups, such as hydroxyls (–OH), carboxyls (–COOH), sulfhydryls (–SH), and amines (–NH$_2$), decrease the partition coefficient of a drug

(e) Hydrophobic groups, such as benzene rings and alkyl (–CH$_3$) groups, increase the partition coefficient

2. Ionization

(a) Drugs that are weak acids and bases can change their pharmacokinetics based on changes in pH

(b) Weak acids dissociate their protons at high pH and become negatively charged, but at low pH they become protonated and carry a neutral charge

(c) Conversely, because weak bases become protonated at low pH, they carry a positive charge at low pH, and at high pH they are neutral because they dissociate their protons

(d) pK$_a$

(1) A drug's pK$_a$ represents the pH at which a given drug will be 50% ionized and 50% un-ionized

(2) For acids, which are neutral at low pH but carry a negative ionic charge at high pH, this means at a pH below the drug's pK$_a$ the drug will be mostly neutral, but at a pH above the pK$_a$ the drug will be mostly negatively ionically charged

(3) For bases, which carry a positive ionic charge at low pH but are neutral at high pH, it means the opposite: at a pH below the drug's pK$_a$ the drug will be mostly positively charged, whereas at a pH above the pK$_a$ the drug will be mostly neutral

    (e) **Neutral drugs cross biological membranes much better than charged drugs**

    (f) This leads to the phenomenon of ion trapping

        (1) Manipulation of pH in different tissue compartments can lead to partitioning of drugs in different tissues

        (2) Acidic drugs are protonated and become neutral in the stomach (low pH) and therefore are readily absorbed, but become negatively charged in the bloodstream (higher pH), thereby inhibiting diffusion of the drug out of the bloodstream

        (3) Alkaline drugs are protonated and carry a positive charge in the stomach due to the low pH, and therefore are poorly absorbed from the stomach, but can be absorbed in the intestines (higher pH), where they dissociate their protons and become neutral, more easily crossing biological membranes

        (4) **Alkaline drugs become ion trapped in the urine** (normally slightly acidic) and are easily excreted, whereas acidic drugs may be passively reabsorbed from the urine across the renal tubules because they become protonated and lose their charge

        (5) **It is possible to alkalinize the urine (by giving intravenous bicarbonate) in order to ion trap acidic drugs in the urine,** preventing their reabsorption and enhancing their excretion—for example, this is done for patients with aspirin overdoses

3. Enterohepatic circulation

    (a) All substances absorbed from the intestines enter the hepatic portal system and are immediately delivered to the liver, the so-called first pass effect

    (b) The liver processes these molecules and then releases them into the hepatic vein heading toward the heart, or into the bile

    (c) **Intravenous administration of drugs bypasses the enterohepatic system for one complete circulation**

    (d) Because drugs have time to diffuse out of the bloodstream during circulation, IV administration results in decreased hepatic metabolism of a drug compared to enteral administration

4. CNS drug distribution

    (a) The endothelium that lines cerebral vessels forms tight junctions, creating the blood-brain barrier which limits diffusion of intravascular molecules into the brain

(b) Because of this barrier, entry of a drug to the CNS requires direct diffusion through the endothelial cell membrane or active transport by endothelial cell membrane pumps

(c) **Thus, drugs that penetrate into the CNS are highly lipid-soluble** (i.e., nonionic), and adding ionic moieties to drugs can be a way to limit CNS toxicities by preventing CNS uptake

5. Materno-fetal drug distribution

   (a) Placental membranes separate the fetal circulation from the maternal circulation

   (b) Thus, as with the CNS, lipid-soluble, nonionic agents are capable of diffusing into the fetal circulation, but ionic agents can only enter by transport pumps

H. Drug metabolism

1. Phase I metabolism

   (a) Cytochrome p450 system

      (1) **Converts nonpolar hydrogens into polar hydroxyl groups**:

      Example: Drug-H + NADPH + $O_2 \rightarrow$ Drug-OH + $NADP^+ + OH^-$

      (2) Cytochrome p450 metabolism occurs in the liver

      (3) The p450 enzymes can be induced by some drugs and repressed by others, leading to potential interactions between drugs that are metabolized by p450 and drugs that induce or repress expression of p450 enzymes

      (4) **Because some drugs both induce p450 and are metabolized by it (e.g., alcohol), the metabolism of these drugs varies dramatically, depending on whether the patient has been chronically exposed to the drug or not**—for example, alcoholics can tolerate huge increases in alcohol doses because of maximally induced expression of their p450 enzymes, whereas first-time drinkers become drunk and die from much lower amounts of alcohol

   (b) Other types of phase I metabolism reactions, including reduction of double bonds, hydrolysis of ester bonds, and enzymatic proteases, all split larger molecules into two smaller molecules

2. Phase II metabolism

   (a) **Conjugation reactions link mildly polar breakdown products of the phase I reactions to much more polar compounds,** allowing the more polar product to be excreted via the urine or bile

   (b) Linkage to highly polar glucuronic acid by the hepatic enzyme glucuronyl transferase is a common mechanism

I. Drug excretion

   1. The kidney is the dominant pathway of drug excretion

   2. The bile excretes small, polar molecules

   3. The **lung is capable of excreting volatile substances by gas diffusion,** particularly nonmetabolizable organic compounds

III. Pharmacodynamics

A. Pharmacodynamics is the drug-receptor interaction and the biological response generated—**pharmacodynam ics is what the drug does to the body**

B. Dissociation constant = K_d

   1. K_d represents the concentration (molarity) of drug at which half the receptors mediating the biological effect are bound, or in biological terms, **the concentration of drug that mediates half the maximum achievable biological response** (see Figure 1.1)

   2. Each individual drug has a K_d, which describes its relationship with a single type of receptor

   3. K_d is also referred to as the "affinity constant," because it represents a measure of the tightness of binding between a drug and its receptor

   4. **Lower K_ds indicate a higher affinity between the drug and the receptor**

      (a) Assume drug X has a K_d of 10^{-5} for receptor 1 (R1) but a K_d of 10^{-8} for receptor 2 (R2)

      (b) This means when drug X is present at 10^{-8} molar, it binds to half of the R2s, but it must be present at 1000-fold higher concentration (10^{-5} molar) to bind half of the R1s—so drug X binds to R2 1000-fold more avidly than to R1

C. Therapeutic index (see Figure 1.4)

   1. Drugs have dose ranges where they are maximally effective and dose ranges where they are maximally toxic

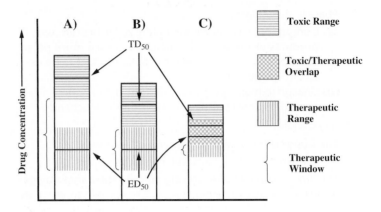

Figure 1.4 Efficacy versus Toxicity
A. An ideal drug has a large interval between the dose that achieves the maximum therapeutic effect and the lowest dose that causes adverse effects. The interval between the lowest therapeutic dose and the lowest toxic dose is called the "therapeutic window." The ED_{50} (effective dose, 50%) of a drug is the concentration at which 50% of maximum efficacy occurs. The TD_{50} (toxic dose, 50%) is the concentration at which 50% of maximum toxicity occurs. **B.** This column depicts a less ideal drug in which there is no cushion between the maximum therapeutic dose and the minimum toxic dose, yet there is no overlap either. Note the narrowed gap between the TD_{50} and the ED_{50}, and the shrinking of the therapeutic window. **C.** An unfortunate reality among drugs is that often the therapeutic doses are the same as the toxic doses. In other words, to get benefit from a drug, people have to put up with side effects. Digoxin, for example, can cause toxicity at almost any dose, but is still widely used in heart failure and atrial fibrillation because of its efficacy.

2. Ideal drugs have effective dose ranges well below their toxic ranges; however, the toxic ranges of many drugs overlap their effective ranges
3. **A drug's therapeutic window is the effective dose range that does not overlap with the toxic dose range**
4. **A drug's therapeutic index is the ratio of the median toxic dose (TD_{50}) to the median effective dose (ED_{50})**

2. AUTONOMIC PHARMACOLOGY

I. Autonomic Physiology

A. Cholinergic agents

1. Acetylcholine binds to two kinds of receptors in the body, nicotinic and muscarinic (see Table 2.1)

2. Muscarinic receptor ligation activates Gq protein → activates phospholipase C (PLC) → ↑ diacylglycerol (DAG) and IP_3 levels → DAG activates protein kinase C (PKC) and IP_3 stimulates calcium release from endoplasmic reticulum → smooth muscle contraction

B. Adrenergic agents

1. There are four types of adrenergic receptors in the body (see Table 2.2)

2. Like muscarinic receptors, all adrenergic receptors use G-proteins as 2nd messengers

3. α-receptors

    (a) α_1-receptor ligation works like muscarinic receptors, via Gq activation of phospholipase C

    (b) α_2-receptor ligation → $G_{inhibitory}$ (G_I)-protein activation → ↓ adenylyl cyclase → ↓ cAMP → ↓ release of presynaptic neurotransmitters

Table 2.1 Cholinergic Receptors

	Nicotinic Receptor	Muscarinic Receptor
Location	Skeletal muscle Postganglionic autonomic neurons	Visceral smooth muscle
Agonists	Acetylcholine Nicotine	Acetylcholine Muscarine Bethanechol
Antagonists	Curare	Atropine

4. β-receptors
    (a) β_1- or β_2-receptor ligation → G_S-protein activation → ↑ adenylyl cyclase → ↑cAMP → PKA → phosphorylation of intracellular proteins → cellular effects
    (b) β-receptor ligation → ↑cardiac contractility, smooth muscle relaxation, ↑ cardiac conduction & automaticity, ↑ glycogenolysis, ↑ lipolysis, ↑ renin secretion (see Table 2.3)
    (c) In general, epinephrine binds to β_1- and β_2-receptors with higher affinity than norepinephrine, but norepinephrine binds to α_1- and α_2-receptors with higher affinity than epinephrine

C. Parasympathetic nervous system (see Figure 2.1)
    1. Uses "cholinergic" neurons, which release acetylcholine at the nerve terminus
    2. Preganglionic parasympathetic fibers synapse in ganglia with postganglionic fibers, which utilize nicotinic receptors to bind to the acetylcholine
    3. Postganglionic fibers synapse with viscera, which utilize muscarinic receptors to bind to acetylcholine
    4. Cholinergic signaling can be clinically manipulated at three major steps (see Figure 2.2)
        (a) Signaling is inhibited by botulinum toxin, which prevents presynaptic release of acetylcholine

---

Figure 2.1 Autonomic Nervous System
Whereas somatic neurons synapse with skeletal muscle and use acetylcholine to signal to postsynaptic nicotinic receptors, autonomic neurons synapse twice before signaling peripheral actions. The first synapse occurs in peripheral ganglia, in which acetylcholine is always used to signal nicotinic receptors on the postsynaptic neurons. The second synapse (the "peripheral synapse") occurs between postganglionic fibers and the viscera. All parasympathetic peripheral synapses use acetylcholine to signal postsynaptic muscarinic receptors. There are three versions of sympathetic visceral synapses. Most viscera receive signals from peripheral sympathetic neurons that secrete norepinephrine, which binds to postsynaptic α- or β-adrenergic receptors. Sweat glands receive signals from peripheral sympathetic neurons that secrete acetylcholine, which binds to post-synaptic muscarinic receptors just like it does to parasympathetic peripheral synapses. Finally, the adrenal medulla does not have a true peripheral synapse; it only has a ganglionic synapse, which uses acetylcholine to signal postsynaptic nicotinic receptors. All ganglionic synapses, including the sympathetic synapse in the adrenal medulla, use acetylcholine to signal nicotinic receptors, and all ganglionic synapses can be blocked with hexamethonium or trimethaphan. Thus, hexamethonium and trimethaphan can completely block parasympathetic and sympathetic signaling in the body.

CNS Neuron	Ganglia	Peripheral Synapse	Tissue	Receptors in Peripheral Synapse — Activation	Receptors in Peripheral Synapse — Inhibition
Somatic		acetylcholine → nicotinic receptor	skeletal muscle	acetylcholine or nicotine	tubocurarine
Parasympathetic	acetylcholine → nicotinic receptor	acetylcholine → muscarinic receptor	smooth muscle, heart, glands	acetylcholine or muscarine	atrophine
Sympathetic #1	acetylcholine → nicotinic receptor	norepinephrine → α & β adrenergic receptor	smooth muscle, heart, glands	norepinephrine or epinephrine	α: phentolamine β: propranolol
Sympathetic #2	acetylcholine → nicotinic receptor	acetylcholine → muscarinic receptor	sweat glands	acetylocholine or muscarine	atrophine
Sympathetic #3	acetylcholine → nicotinic receptor	norepinephrine epinephrine	adrenal medulla	**Ganglia Activation:** acetylcholie or nicotine	**Ganglia Inhibition:** hexamethonium or trimethaphan

15

Table 2.2 Adrenergic Receptors

	α_1	α_2	β_1	β_2
Location	Smooth muscle	Presynaptic nerve terminals	Smooth muscle Heart	Smooth muscle Bronchioles
Effects	• Smooth muscle contract • Vasoconstrict • ↑ BP • Mydriasis	• ↓ Norepi-nephrine release from presynaptic terminal	• Smooth muscle contract • ↑ HR • ↑ Cardiac contractility	• Smooth muscle relax • ↓ BP • Bronchodilate
Agonists	norepinephrine phenylephrine dopamine epinephrine	norepinephrine clonidine tizanidine epinephrine	norepinephrine epinephrine isoproterenol dopamine dobutamine	epinephrine isoproterenol
Antagonists	prazosin terazosin doxazosin phentolamine labetalol	phentolamine	labetalol propranolol metoprolol atenolol betaxolol carvedilol	labetalol propranolol carvedilol

Table 2.3 Autonomic Effect on Organs

Organ	Sympathetic Input	Parasympathetic Input
Heart	↑ HR ↑ Contractile force ↑ Automaticity	↓ HR ↓ Automaticity
Vasculature	NE → Vasoconstrict, ↑ BP Epi → Vasodilate skeletal muscle beds	Minimal innervation
Eye	Mydriasis (radial muscle contraction) **No effect on accommodation at all!!!**	Miosis (circular muscle contraction) Accommodation for near vision (ciliary muscle contraction)
GI	↓ Motility/tone ⊕ sphincter contraction	↑ Motility/tone
Salivary glands	↑ Viscous saliva	↑↑↑ Watery saliva
Sweat glands	↑ Sweat	No effect

(b) Signaling is stimulated by inhibition of acetylcholinesterase, which normally degrades acetylcholine in the synaptic cleft—blockade of this enzyme prolongs the life of acetylcholine, thereby increasing signaling

(c) Signaling can be directly induced by administration of cholinomimetics and inhibited by cholinolytics, which are chemically similar to acetylcholine and therefore bind to its receptor

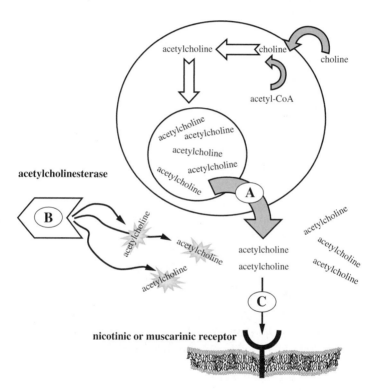

Figure 2.2 Cholinergic Synapse
Acetylcholine is formed in the presynaptic nerve terminus by linkage of acetyl-CoA to choline. **A.** The acetylcholine is stored in vesicles that fuse with the cell membrane at the nerve terminus when the nerve is depolarized. Botulinum toxin inhibits this vesicular release of acetylcholine. **B.** Acetylcholine in the synaptic cleft continues to signal its postsynaptic receptor until the acetylcholine is degraded by the enzyme acetylcholinesterase. Acetylcholinesterase is the dominant regulator of the duration of cholinergic signaling. Inhibition of acetylcholinesterase is a major method by which clinicians intervene to promote parasympathetic responses. **C.** Postsynaptic nicotinic or muscarinic receptor antagonists and direct agonists are also widely used in medicine.

D. Sympathetic nervous system (see Figure 2.1)

1. Like parasympathetic neurons, all preganglionic sympathetic neurons secrete acetylcholine at the nerve terminus

2. There are three kinds of sympathetic synapses with peripheral organs

   (a) Postganglionic sympathetic neurons synapsing with visceral organs secrete norepinephrine to transmit signals to α- and β-adrenergic receptors on the visceral organs

   (b) Postganglionic sympathetic neurons synapsing with sweat glands secrete acetylcholine to transmit signals to muscarinic receptors on the sweat glands

   (c) Preganglionic sympathetic neurons synapsing with the adrenal medulla secrete acetylcholine to transmit signals to nicotinic receptors on the adrenal medulla (Note: there is no postganglionic fiber in this pathway, as the preganglionic fiber synapses directly with the adrenal medulla)

3. Adrenergic signaling can be clinically manipulated at eight major steps (see Figure 2.3)

E. Predominant autonomic tone (see Table 2.4)

1. **In most organs, parasympathetic innervation dominates over sympathetic signals at baseline**

2. Pharmacologic blockade of autonomic ganglia (simultaneous blocking of sympathetic and parasympathetic ganglia) thus tends to lead to sympathetic-like responses in the organs

F. Autonomic reflexes

1. **Autonomic signaling in the viscera tends to maintain cardiovascular homeostasis**

   (a) Interventions causing vasoconstriction lead to reflex bradycardia in order to maintain a homeostatic blood pressure, and interventions causing vasodilation lead to reflex tachycardia

   (b) Conversely, interventions that directly increase heart rate cause a reflex vasodilation to maintain blood pressure, and interventions that slow the heart rate cause reflex vasoconstriction

   (c) The carotid body is the major blood pressure sensor in the autonomic nervous system, and it directly mediates autonomic reflexes affecting the heart and the vasculature depending on changes in the blood pressure

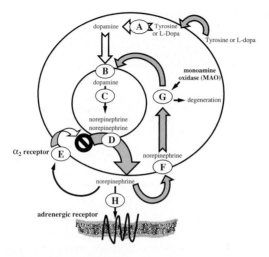

Figure 2.3 Adrenergic Synapse

A. After tyrosine and L-dopa are imported into the presynaptic nerve terminus, they are converted to dopamine via the action of tyrosine hydroxylase. This is the rate-limiting step in the synthesis of norepinephrine, and this step can be blocked with the adrenolytic agent metyrosine. **B.** After dopamine is formed in the cytosol of the presynaptic nerve terminus, it is pumped into storage vesicles. In addition, norepinephrine taken up into the presynaptic nerve terminus can also be pumped into the storage vesicles. The adrenolytics reserpine and guanethidine can block this vesicular transport pump. **C.** Once inside the storage vesicle, dopamine is converted to norepinephrine by the enzyme dopamine decarboxylase. The adrenolytic α-methyldopa can act as a false substrate to dopamine decarboxylase, competitively inhibiting formation of norepinephrine.

D. Depolarization of the nerve terminus causes the storage vesicles to fuse with the plasma membrane at the nerve terminus, thereby releasing norepinephrine into the synaptic cleft. Multiple drugs affect this step. The sympathomimetics tyrosine, amphetamines, ephedrine, and pseudoephedrine all stimulate release of norepinephrine from the storage vesicles. The adrenolytic guanethidine stabilizes the presynaptic plasma membrane, preventing vesicle fusion with the nerve terminus (although initially guanethidine has some mild tyramine-like properties that can cause a brief increase in norepinephrine release prior to inhibition).

E. Norepinephrine in the synaptic cleft normally ligates the presynaptic α_2-receptor, which feedback-inhibits further vesicular release of norepinephrine. Clonidine, guanabenz, and α-methyldopa also ligate the α_2-receptor, inhibiting norepinephrine release. **F.** Catecholamines remaining in the synaptic cleft after spillage can be taken back up into the presynaptic nerve terminus. Cocaine acts as a sympathomimetic by inhibiting reuptake of catecholamines in the synaptic cleft, leading to prolonged signaling. The adrenolytic guanethidine also mediates a temporary initial block of reuptake of catecholamines. **G.** Inhibitors of monoamine oxidase block the degradation of norepinephrine. These drugs are not useful as sympathomimetics, however, as they only increase levels of catecholamines within the nerve terminus, not in the synaptic cleft where signaling occurs. **H.** Finally, postsynaptic α- and β-receptors are amenable to direct agonism with pressor agents or direct antagonism with adrenergic blockers.

Table 2.4 Predominant Autonomic Tone

Organ	Baseline Tone	Effect of Ganglionic Blockade
Heart	↓ HR	↑ HR
Vasculature	Vasoconstriction (↑ BP)	Vasodilation (↓ BP)
Lung	Bronchoconstriction	Bronchodilation
GI	Slow motility	Fast motility
Sweat glands	↑ Sweat (↓ core temperature)	↓ Sweat (↑ core temperature)

2. A classic clinical example of autonomic reflex is the use of vasodilators to decrease blood pressure, which may have detrimental effects on ischemic myocardium by causing a reflex increase in heart rate, thereby increasing myocardial oxygen demand

II. Cholinomimetics (see Table 2.5)

A. There are two classes of cholinomimetics: direct receptor agonists and inhibitors of acetylcholinesterase

B. Direct receptor agonists are designed to be chemically resistant to degradation by acetylcholinesterase, thus leading to prolonged receptor signaling following administration

C. Acetylcholinesterase inhibitors

1. Three classes

   (a) **Competitive reversible inhibitors are used for diagnosis of myasthenia gravis and are very short-acting—** administration leads to rapid improvement in strength of myasthenia patients due to improved acetylcholine signaling at neuromuscular junctions

   (b) Poor enzyme substrates are called "carbamates"

   (1) **They last longer and are therefore useful for therapeutics**

   (2) Used to treat myasthenia gravis, and new drugs, donepezil and galantamine, are used to treat Alzheimer's; they slow cognitive decline by increasing acetylcholine in the brain

Table 2.5 Cholinomimetics

Durg	Characteristics	Use
Direct Receptor Agonists		
bethanechol *musc ®* *- Ach related*	• Carries a positive charge → ↓ CNS penetration • Not degraded by acetylcholinesterase	Stimulates *⊕ intest.* urination in pts with neurogenic bladder
Acetylcholinesterase Inhibitors		
pilocarpine *⊕ sweat, tears, saliva*	• Uncharged/lipophilic → ↑ CNS penetration • Able to penetrate cornea if applied topically • Not degraded by acetylcholinesterase	Topical eye drop → miosis → open Schlemm's canal → ↓ pressure in glaucoma
edrophonium	• A reversible inhibitor, short-acting	Dx-myasthenia gravis
neostigmine	• Carbamate (poor acetylcholinesterase substrate) • Quaternary ammonium compound so carries positive charge; does not penetrate CNS	Tx-myasthenia gravis
pyridostigmine	• Carbamate (poor acetylcholinesterase substrate) • Quaternary ammonium compound; does not penetrate CNS	Tx-myasthenia gravis *- long-acting*
physostigmine	• Carbamate (poor acetylcholinesterase substrate) • Tertiary amine; does not carry positive charge and does penetrate CNS	Eye drops → miosis → lower intraocular pressure in glaucoma
donepezil & galantamine	• Carbamate (poor acetylcholinesterase substrate); good CNS penetration • Good CNS penetration	Increase acetylcholine levels in CNS, slow cognitive decline in Alzheimer's

AUTONOMIC PHARMACOLOGY

(*Continued*)

Table 2.5 (Continued)

Durg	Characteristics	Use
	Acetylcholinesterase Inhibitors	
malathion	• Organophosphate (irreversible inhibitor) • Requires metabolic activation for full effect, and this activation selectively occurs in insect cells, making the drug much more toxic for insects than humans	Insecticide
sarin	• Organophosphate (irreversible inhibitor) • Undergoes very rapid aging	Chemical warfare

    (c) Irreversible inhibitors

        (1) These drugs are called "organophosphates"

        (2) They form covalent bonds with the active site of acetylcholinesterase, irreversibly blocking the enzyme's activity

        (3) Organophosphates are useful as pesticides or chemical warfare agents

  2. Toxicity is caused by ingestion or direct skin contact with organophosphates (irreversible inhibitors)

    (a) Presents with hypercholinergic signs and symptoms, including hypersecretion of saliva and mucus, bronchospasm, miosis, bradycardia, vomiting, diarrhea

    (b) **Pralidoxime is the principal antidote for organophosphate toxicity**

        (1) It splits the covalent bond between the organophosphate and acetylcholinesterase, thereby regenerating the enzyme

        (2) The bond between the organophosphate and acetylcholinesterase is somewhat unstable, and over time chemically changes, a process called "aging"

        (3) **Pralidoxime is incapable of breaking the bond once it has aged,** and thus pralidoxime must be administered quickly after organophosphate toxicity or it will not be effective

(4) Atropine (see section III, Cholinolytics) is a muscarinic antagonist that can be used to treat the cholinomimetic symptoms of organophosphate toxicity, but because of its transient effects, it is not curative

III. Cholinolytics

A. Come in three varieties, muscarinic receptor antagonists, ganglionic blockers (nicotinic receptor antagonists), and neuromuscular blocking agents (a subtype of nicotinic antagonists)

B. Muscarinic antagonists (see Table 2.6)

1. Atropine is the most familiar drug in this class

2. Toxicity of muscarinic antagonists causes the well-known syndrome of: **dry as a bone** (no saliva, sweat, or urine), **mad as a hatter** (confusion/delirium), **hot as a hare** (increased core temperature), **blind as a bat** (mydriasis and cycloplegia = lack of accommodation)

C. Ganglionic blockers (see Table 2.6)

1. Affect peripheral parasympathetic nerve synapses and ganglionic synapses in both the sympathetic and parasympathetic pathways—skeletal muscle nicotinic receptors are slightly different than autonomic nicotinic receptors, so ganglionic blockers are much less potent at blocking nicotinic receptors in somatic skeletal muscle synapses (see Figure 2.1)

Table 2.6 Muscarinic and Ganglionic Blockers

Drug	Characteristics & Uses
Muscarinic Antagonists	
atropine	• Used for bradycardia, for heart block, and to reverse cholinergic poisoning
benztropine	• Penetrates CNS well, used for Parkinson's dz, by ↓ cholinergic signaling, helps restore the cholinergic/dopaminergic balance in the brain
cyclopentolate	• Topical eyedrops → ciliary paralysis → mydriasis → allows funduscopic examination, but also inhibits accommodation → ↓ near vision
ipratropium	• Used as an inhaler to bronchodilate asthma patients
oxybutynin	• Used as a urinary stimulant for neurogenic bladder
scopolamine	• Used orally or topically as a remedy for motion sickness

(Continued)

Table 2.6 (Continued)

Drug	Characteristics & Uses
trihexyphenidyl	• Like benztropine, can be used for Parkinson's dz, penetrates CNS well
	Ganglionic Blockers
trimethaphan	• Used for hypertensive emergencies where rapid, titratable IV dosing allows for complete control of blood pressure
	• Short half-life means changes in IV infusion rate lead to rapid changes in serum levels, allowing rapid titration to blood pressure changes
	• Does not cross CNS
mecamylamine	• Rarely used clinically; similar to trimethaphan except penetrates CNS

2. Thus, these drugs completely abrogate autonomic signaling in the body but relatively spare skeletal muscle, leading to reversion to predominant autonomic tone (see Table 2.4) → mydriasis with loss of accommodation, tachycardia, hypotension, constipation, urinary retention

D. Neuromuscular blocking agents (see Table 2.7)

1. Principally used for anesthesia and intubation of patients in emergencies

2. Unlike ganglionic agents, these drugs are much more potent at blocking skeletal muscle nicotinic receptors than autonomic receptors

3. Come in two varieties, depolarizing and nondepolarizing

   (a) Depolarizing agents

   (1) Bind to acetylcholine receptors and act as partial agonists, which leads to refractoriness of receptor signaling

   (2) Cause fasciculations at first due to depolarization

   (3) **Due to intense muscle contraction at first, depolarizing agents may cause hyperkalemia and should be avoided in patients with hyperkalemia, renal failure, burns, rhabdomyolysis, or any condition associated with hyperkalemia**

   (b) Nondepolarizing agents act as competitive antagonists of acetylcholine receptors

4. Both varieties cause complete paralysis of voluntary muscles

Table 2.7 Neuromuscular Blockers

Drug	Duration	Characteristics
		Depolarizing Agent
succinyl-choline	2–4 min	• Very rapid onset (1–2 min) & duration • Useful for rapid sequence intubation in emergencies • Causes muscular fibrillation, can cause hyperkalemia • Some pts have enzyme polymorphism → slow metabolism of succinylcholine; these pts have paralysis for hours
		Nondepolarizing Agents
tubocurarine	<60 min	• Prototype drug, long duration of action • Causes ↓ BP due to ganglionic blockade and histamine release
pancuronium	<60 min	• Long duration of effect, may cause tachy-cardia
atracurium	15 min	• Spontaneously decomposes in plasma, so not renally cleared • Drug of choice in patients with renal or hepatic failure • Can cause histamine-associated hypotension
vecuronium	30 min	• Cleared by liver, avoid in hepatic failure • No cardiovascular side effects, drug of choice in pts with cardiovascular disease or hypotensive
rocuronium	30 min	• New drug • Very rapid onset (1–2 min), similar to succinylcholine • No cardiovascular side effects

Handwritten annotations: contracts muscle 1st → twitching → flaccid paralysis; blocks N_M; intubation

IV. Sympathomimetics (Adrenomimetics)

A. There are three classes of sympathomimetics: direct agonists, indirect agonists, & mixed agonists

B. Direct adrenergic agonists bind to α- or β-receptors (see Table 2.8)

C. **Indirect adrenergic agonists increase the level of norepinephrine in the synaptic cleft** (see Table 2.9)

1. Some increase the release of transmitter from the presynaptic terminus
2. Some decrease the reuptake or degradation of norepinephrine in the synaptic cleft

D. Mixed agonists bind to receptors and increase the level of norepinephrine in the synaptic cleft (see Tables 2.8 & 2.9)

Table 2.8 Sympathomimetics: Direct Adrenergic Agonists

Drug	Receptors	Characteristics
epinephrine	$\alpha_1\alpha_2\beta_1\beta_2$	• $\beta_2 \rightarrow$ vasodilation in skeletal muscle beds—note that at high concentrations (such as those used during code blue), α effects dominate, epinephrine $\rightarrow$ vasoconstriction $\rightarrow \uparrow$ BP
		• $\beta_1 \rightarrow \uparrow$ cardiac contractility, $\uparrow$ HR; $\beta_2 \rightarrow$ bronchodilation *ER asthma*
		• $\beta_1 \rightarrow \uparrow$ glycogenolysis & gluconeogenesis in liver, $\uparrow$ insulin production, $\uparrow$ skeletal muscle uptake of glucose
		• 1st line for anaphylactic shock & cardiac resuscitation
norepinephrine	$\alpha_1\alpha_2\beta_1$	• $\alpha_1 \rightarrow$ vasoconstrict, no β_2 activity to counteract α_1 effects
		• $\beta_1 \rightarrow \uparrow$ contractility, $\uparrow$ HR
		• In normotensive animals, norepinephrine causes reflex bradycardia 2° to induction of profound hypertension, which overwhelms its less potent direct β_1 effect
		• In hypotensive patients, norepinephrine increases the BP toward normal but not above, so there is no reflex bradycardia, and the direct β_1 effect causes tachycardia, which can precipitate or worsen myocardial ischemia
ephedrine	$\alpha_1\alpha_2\beta_1\beta_2$	• A mixed agonist, weak direct agonism for all receptors
		• Most of efficacy is from indirect agonism (see Table 2.9)

Table 2.8 (Continued)

Drug	Receptors	Characteristics
pseudoephedrine	$\alpha_1\alpha_2\beta_1\beta_2$	• Levo-stereoisomer of ephedrine, also a mixed agonist • Most of efficacy is from indirect agonism (see Table 2.9)
isoproterenol	$\beta_1\beta_2$	• β-selective agonist • $\beta_1 \to$ ↑ contractility & ↑ HR • $\beta_2 \to$ vasodilation & ↓ BP, bronchodilation • Dominant cardiovascular effect is marked widening of the pulse pressure due to ↑ systolic BP from ↑ cardiac output, but ↓ diastolic BP from direct and reflex vasodilation
dopamine	$\alpha_1\beta_1$	• 1st-line pressor for most clinical conditions • $\alpha_1 \to$ ↑ vasoconstriction, ↑ BP; $\beta_1 \to$ ↑ contractility, ↑ HR • Vasoconstriction of pulmonary arteries may blunt the ↑ cardiac output effects stimulated by dopamine, so in pts with poor ejection fractions, dobutamine may be a better option • Specific dopamine receptors also cause renal artery dilation, which may promote diuresis
dobutamine	β_1	• $\beta_1 \to$ ↑ contractility, ↑ HR • Agent of choice in patients with heart failure • May cause reflexive vasodilation from ↑ cardiac output, which can ↓ BP • Can be mixed with dopamine to simultaneously improve cardiac output and prevent reflexive vasodilation

shock

(Continued)

Table 2.8 (Continued)

Drug	Receptors	Characteristics
phenylephrine	α_1	• $\alpha_1 \rightarrow$ vasoconstriction, ↑ BP • Autonomic reflex ↓ HR due to ↑ BP and lack of β_1 agonism • Useful pressor for pts with tachycardia or ischemia • Also useful as a topical eyedrop to stimulate mydriasis for funduscopic exams and as a nasal decongestant by causing vasoconstriction of nasal vasculature $\rightarrow$ ↓ mucosal edema • **Note that unlike cholinolytic drugs, phenylephrine causes mydriasis without cycloplegia (inhibition of accommodation) because it has no effect on ciliary muscle**
albuterol	β_2	• Selective β_2 agonist, used as an inhaled bronchodilator • At high doses $\rightarrow$ systemic absorption $\rightarrow$ vasodilation and reflex tachycardia
salmeterol	β_2	• Longer acting albuterol-like agent, useful for asthma
mirtazapine	α_2	• Selective α_2 antagonist, antidepressant (see Tables 2.9 & 3.5)
oxymetazoline	$\alpha_1\alpha_2$	• α_1 agonist, vasoconstriction for nasal congestion • Rebound congestion after prolonged use and addiction potential

E. **Note that not all drugs with direct agonism for adrenergic receptors are sympathomimetics**—for example, clonidine and tizanidine directly agonize the α_2-receptor; however, because α_2-ligation inhibits adrenergic signaling, they are considered adrenolytics

F. **Understanding the effects of sympathomimetics on the host cardiovascular system is the key to answering test questions about autonomic consequences of pharmacologic intervention** (see Figure 2.4 & Table 2.10)

1. Norepinephrine

(a) **The dominant physiologic effect of norepinephrine is profound α_1-mediated vasoconstriction,** causing a marked increase in both systolic and diastolic blood pressure

Table 2.9 Sympathomimetics: Indirect Adrenergic Agonists

Drug	Characteristics
tyramine	• A normal byproduct of tyrosine metabolism, also found at high concentrations in fermented foods, e.g., wine & cheese • Degraded by MAO in presynaptic nerve terminus • Causes release of stored norepinephrine (Figure 2.3D), effects mimic direct administration of norepinephrine • Pts taking MAO inhibitors who ingest tyramine can develop severe ↑ BP
amphetamine	• Highly lipophilic with potent CNS effects • Stimulates release of catecholamines (Figure 2.3D) • Methamphetamine is a derivative with even more potent CNS activity • Methylphenidate is a derivative used to Tx attention deficit disorder, narcolepsy
sibutramine	• A substituted amphetamine that promotes weight loss by suppressing appetite; blocks reuptake of serotonin and NE in CNS
atomoxetine	• Selective NE reuptake inhibitor for attention deficit disorder
duloxetine	• Novel antidepressant works by inhibiting CNS reuptake of serotonin and NE
mirtazapine	• Presynaptic α_2 antagonism results in increased release of NE
ephedrine	• Dominant effect is stimulate release of catecholamines (Figure 2.3D) • Also has weak, direct agonism properties • Overall effects most closely mimic epinephrine (contrast with tyramine) • Highly lipophilic so has CNS effects • Found at low doses in cough syrups and decongestants
pseudoephedrine	• The levo-isomer of ephedrine, it has minimal CNS effects • Same mechanism as ephedrine • Used as decongestant: vasoconstriction → ↓ mucosal edema

(Continued)

Table 2.9 (Continued)

Drug	Characteristics
	• Eyedrops → mydriasis, used for funduscopic examination • Contraindicated in patients with coronary disease, as it can precipitate hypertension if systemically absorbed
cocaine	• Highly lipophilic, thus potent CNS effects • Inhibits reuptake of catecholamines in the synaptic cleft (Figure 2.3F) • Leads to prolonged stimulation of CNS adrenergic neurons
MAO Inhibitors (MAOIs)	• Include selegiline (irreversible inhibition of MAO subtype B, which is only found in the CNS), phenelzine, and tranylcypromine • Mostly affect CNS neurons • Have anticholinergic effects and serotonin-stimulatory effects, but minimal pressor effects unless mixed with high doses of tyramine

  (b) **In normotensive hosts, the ↑ systemic vascular resistance and ↑ BP → autonomic reflex bradycardia, which overwhelms norepinephrine's less potent agonism of β_1-receptors on the heart (which would otherwise cause tachycardia)**
  (c) **In hypotensive patients there is no reflex bradycardia seen when norepinephrine is used as a pressor** because the overall effect is to bring BP back toward normal rather than to increase it above normal, and thus in these patients norepinephrine's direct β_1 agonism is unopposed, leading to pressor-induced tachycardia, a common side effect of norepinephrine in hypotensive patients
 2. Epinephrine
  (a) **Epinephrine causes a predominant increase in myocardial contractility and heart rate because of β_1 and β_2 agonism**
  (b) Normotensive hosts
   (1) The increase in cardiac output leads to a reflex vasodilation, which decreases systemic vascular resistance (SVR)

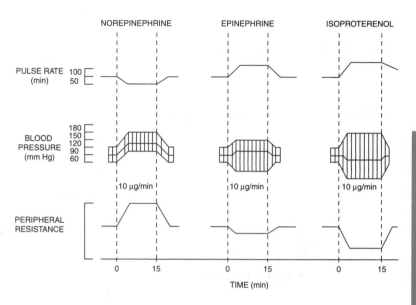

Figure 2.4 Hemodynamic Effects of Catecholamines

A. Norepinephrine causes a dominant α_1-mediated vasoconstriction, leading to increased systemic vascular resistance and hence increased blood pressure. The carotid bodies sense this increased blood pressure and mediate a cholinergic reflex to slow the pulse in an attempt to return the blood pressure to baseline. The cholinergic reflex overwhelms the direct effect of norepinephrine on the β_1-receptors of the heart. Note that this reflex is NOT intact in a hypotensive patient, because the use of norepinephrine as a pressor in such a patient moves the blood pressure TOWARD homeostasis (toward normal), rather than above normal. **B.** Epinephrine causes more potent direct β_1-agonism than does norepinephrine, and hence increased heart rate and contractility, which increases cardiac output. However, β_2 agonism caused by epinephrine leads to peripheral vasodilation, an effect potentiated by the carotid bodies, which sense the increased cardiac output and cause a reflex vasodilation to return the blood pressure toward normal. The overall effect is a widening of the pulse pressure, with the systolic blood pressure increased by the increased cardiac output, but the diastolic blood pressure reduced from peripheral vasodilation. **C.** Isoproterenol lacks any α_1 signaling. Thus, like epinephrine, there is an increased pulse pressure due to β_1-mediated increased cardiac output. Although epinephrine does mediate some α_1 effect, isoproterenol does not, so the pulse pressure is widened even more than for epinephrine because there is no direct vasoconstriction to counteract the β_2-mediated vasodilation and reflex vasodilation mediated by the carotid bodies.

Table 2.10 Effects of Sympathomimetics in Normotensive Subjects

Drug	HR	SBP	DBP	SVR	Comments
norepinephrine	↓	↑↑	↑↑	↑↑	• Dominant effect is ↑ BP • Reflex ↓ HR
epinephrine	↑	↑	↓	↓	• Dominant effect is ↑ contractility & HR • Reflexive ↓ SVR & BP • Note widened pulse pressure
isoproterenol	↑	↑	↓↓	↓↓	• Dominant effect is ↑ HR & contractility, ↓ SVR • Reflexes less important; markedly ↑ pulse pressure

SBP = systolic blood pressure, DBP = diastolic blood pressure, SVR = systemic vascular resistance

      (2) Because cardiac output is increased, the systolic pressure goes up despite the lowered SVR, but the lowered SVR results in lower diastolic pressure—**the overall effect is a widening of the pulse pressure**

      (3) The direct α_1 vasoconstriction and β_2 vasodilation antagonize each other and are overwhelmed by the reflex autonomic response

    (c) In hypotensive patients, when epinephrine is used at high doses it causes direct vasoconstriction (α_1 effect), bronchodilation, and increased contractility and heart rate

3. Isoproterenol

    (a) **Causes ↑ HR and contractility from β_1 agonism, and ↓ SVR from β_2 agonism**

    (b) Because the ↑ cardiac output 2° to ↑ HR/contractility is directly opposed by the ↓ SVR, there is little effect attributable to autonomic reflex—in essence, isoproterenol mediates two opposing effects on BP, and little autonomic reflex is involved

    (c) **The overall result is a marked widening of the pulse pressure** with typically a slight ↓ overall mean arterial pressure—↑ systolic BP but ↓ diastolic BP

(d) Isoproterenol is less commonly used clinically as a pressor because of this propensity to decrease mean arterial pressure

V. Adrenolytics

A. Inhibit adrenergic signaling

B. These drugs have multiple mechanisms, affecting synthesis or release of catecholamines from the presynaptic nerve terminus, or direct postsynaptic receptor antagonism (see Figure 2.3)

C. Three general classes

1. Inhibitors of presynaptic adrenergic signaling (see Table 2.11)

   (a) Inhibit the synthesis, storage, or release of catecholamines from the presynaptic nerve terminus

   (b) Rarely used for antihypertension because of CNS depression and other toxicity, but tizanidine is a new drug that improves muscle spasticity in patients with multiple sclerosis or spinal cord injury

   (c) **The only 1st-line hypertension indication for any of these drugs is the use of α-methyldopa as an antihypertensive in pregnant women**

2. Inhibitors of postsynaptic α_1-receptors: α-blockers (see Table 2.12)

   (a) **These drugs cause marked reflex tachycardia, which limits their usefulness**

   (b) 1st-line indications:

       (1) Phenoxybenzamine and phentolamine for pheochromocytoma-induced hypertension

       (2) **Prazosin, terazosin, doxazosin for hypertension in a patient with benign prostatic hypertrophy (BPH)—** α-blockers relax the bladder–neck detrusor muscle, allowing improved urination in patients with BPH, so patients who are both hypertensive and have BPH can be treated with a single agent

3. Inhibitors of postsynaptic β-receptors: β-blockers (see Table 2.13)

   (a) **Proven to decrease mortality in patients with hypertension**

   (b) **Proven to decrease mortality in patients with myocardial ischemia**

   (c) **Proven to decrease mortality in patients with heart failure**

Table 2.11 Adrenolytics: Synthesis, Storage, & Secretion Inhibitors

Drug	Characteristics
clonidine	• Selective α_2 agonist, inhibits release of norepinephrine from presynaptic terminals (see Figure 2.3E) • Causes vasodilation by suppressing norepinephrine-mediated constriction, and, importantly, does NOT induce reflex tachycardia because the suppression of norepinephrine release blunts the normal autonomic reflex • Useful as an antihypertensive agent in patients with refractory hypertension, particularly in renal failure, and pts withdrawing from illicit drugs • Not 1st line because of side effects (e.g., CNS depression, fatigue, dry mouth)
tizanidine	• α_2 agonist similar to clonidine, muscle relaxant (Table 3.10)
guanabenz	• Similar to clonidine, but rarely used clinically
methyldopa	• Similar to clonidine, but also acts as a partial agonist–antagonist of α_1-receptors and inhibits norepinephrine synthesis by acting as an alternative substrate for dopamine decarboxylase (see Figure 2.3C, E, H) • Because of CNS depressant effects and propensity to cause drug-induced lupus, this drug is rarely used **except in pregnancy**, when it is considered a 1st-line antihypertensive
metyrosine	• Competitively inhibits tyrosine hydroxylase, the rate-limiting enzyme, thus blocking norepinephrine synthesis (see Figure 2.3A) • Severe CNS depression limits its clinical utility
reserpine	• Blocks uptake of dopamine into synaptic vesicles, and blocks reuptake of norepinephrine into synaptic vesicles (see Figure 2.3B) • Prevention of uptake into vesicles leads to degradation of norepinephrine by MAO, causing depletion of synaptic norepinephrine • The drug is rarely used currently due to CNS depression
guanethidine	• Has four separate adrenolytic effects: $\Rightarrow$ Dominant effect is reserpine-like block of uptake into synaptic vesicles (see Figure 2.3B)

Table 2.11 (Continued)

Drug	Characteristics
	⇒ Stabilizes plasma membrane, inhibiting vesicle fusion and thus inhibiting catecholamine release from the presynaptic terminus (see Figure 2.3D)
	⇒ Prior to membrane stabilization, actually has a tyramine-like stimulation of synaptic spilling of norepinephrine, leading to presynaptic depletion of norepinephrine, thus causing an initial INCREASE in blood pressure followed by a decrease (see Figure 2.3D)
	⇒ Exerts a cocaine-like blockade of norepinephrine reuptake into the presynaptic nerve terminus, contributing to an initial INCREASE in blood pressure (see Figure 2.3F)
	• Rarely used clinically

Table 2.12 Adrenolytics: α-Blockers

Drug	Characteristics
phentolamine	• Nonselective competitive inhibitor of α_1- and α_2-receptors
	• Direct effect of α_1 blockade is potent vasodilation → ↓ BP
	• This causes a reflex increase in presynaptic norepinephrine release → β_1 agonism → ↑ HR and renin secretion to maintain homeostatic BP
	• Key concept: because of simultaneous α_2 blockade, there is no feedback inhibition of presynaptic norepinephrine release, and the normal autonomic reflex causing ↑ HR in response to vasodilation is magnified
	• Thus phentolamine causes severe reflex tachycardia and palpitations, and generally must be combined with a β-blocker to prevent this
	• Other side effects include nasal congestion, miosis, and decreased ejaculation from α_1 antagonism, and ↑ GI motility (diarrhea) from α_2 antagonism
	• The drug is used primarily to treat pheochromocytoma-induced ↑ BP
phenoxy-benzamine	• An irreversible inhibitor of α_1- and α_2-receptors
	• Alkylates the receptors, forming covalent bonds with them
	• Acts similarly to phentolamine, rarely used clinically

(Continued)

Table 2.12 (Continued)

Drug	Characteristics
prazosin terazosin doxazosin	• All are selective α_1 antagonists • Because they do not block α_2, they cause much less reflex tachycardia than nonselective inhibitors • However, at the same time, the lack of α_2 blockade allows a blunting of the normal autonomic reflex, which leads to prominent orthostatic hypotension (vasodilation → ↓ BP, when person stands there is an inappropriate lack of ↑ HR, which causes the BP to fall even further) • Although α_1 antagonists can be used as antihypertensives, their use is limited by orthostatic hypotension and also by the moderate reflex tachycardia, which is undesirable in patients who have underlying coronary disease • The chief use of these agents is benign prostatic hypertrophy (BPH), as α_1 blockade relaxes the bladder sphincter → marked improvement in urination—when used as an antihypertensive agent, it is almost always in people who also have BPH, allowing the clinician to treat two diseases with one drug
alfuzosin	• α_1 antagonist, similar to prazosin, but indicated only for benign prostatic hypertrophy • Highly selective for prostate activity, with diminished vascular side effects
carvedilol	• Nonselective α_1- and β_1-, β_2-receptor blocker • See Table 2.12 for properties
labetalol	• Nonselective α_1- and β_1-, β_2-receptor blocker • See Table 2.12 for properties
yohimbine	• Selective α_2 antagonist • Not clinically useful—previously suggested as a therapy for impotence

    (d) 1st-line indications include each of the preceding, as well as rate control in patients with tachyarrhythmias and control of hypertension in aortic dissection

    (e) Also useful for migraine headaches, thyroid storm, tremor, and performance anxiety

Table 2.13 Adrenolytics: β-Blockers

Drug	Receptor	Characteristics
Acebutolol	β_1	• Used for hypertension, qd or bid dosing—po only
Atenolol	β_1	• Used for hypertension, qd or bid dosing—po or IV
Betaxolol	β_1	• Used for hypertension, qd dosing—po only • Most highly β_1 selective of all available drugs • Longest half-life of all β-blockers
Metoprolol	β_1	• Used for hypertension, acute ischemia, heart failure—po or IV • Easiest of the β-blockers to administer IV, making metoprolol the most commonly used agent for patients with acute ischemia • Usually bid dosing, although an extended release form is available
Bisoprolol	β_1	• Used for hypertension and heart failure, qd dosing—po only
Esmolol	β_1	• Extremely short acting, must administer via IV drip—IV only • 1st-line therapy for acute aortic dissection • Also useful for hypertensive emergency or acute supraventricular tachycardias refractory to other therapies
Nadolol	β_1, β_2	• Nonselective β-blocker, rarely used, qd dosing—po only
Pindolol	β_1, β_2	• Nonselective β-blocker, rarely used, bid dosing—po only • Has "intrinsic sympathomimetic activity" (ISA), which means it actually acts as a partial β_2-receptor agonist, making it even less likely to induce bronchospasm in asthmatics
Propranolol	β_1, β_2	• Highly lipophilic, causing more CNS effects than other drugs • Because of CNS effects, propranolol is still used for control of essential tremor or for performance anxiety disorder • Also, because it is the only drug studied in the condition, propranolol is still used as prophylaxis

(Continued)

Table 2.13 (Continued)

Drug	Receptor	Characteristics
		to prevent variceal bleeding in patients with portal hypertension
		• Short acting, dosing typically tid—po only
Timolol	β_1, β_2	• Major use is in eye drops for glaucoma; rarely used for HTN
Labetalol	α_1, β_1, β_2	• Nonselective adrenergic inhibitor, very potent reducer of BP
		• Useful for HTN, hypertensive emergency, aortic dissection
		• Can be dosed po bid or IV for emergencies
		• Like pindolol, labetalol has intrinsic sympathomimetic activity
Carvedilol	α_1, β_1, β_2	• Nonselective adrenergic inhibitor
		• 1st β-blocker proven to reduce mortality in heart failure—1st-line indication for heart failure
		• The ONLY β-blocker that has been proven to reduce mortality in severe (Class IV) heart failure
		• Can be dosed po bid—no IV formulation

(f) Propranolol has been proven to decrease the risk of recurrent variceal bleeding in patients with portal hypertension by decreasing portal pressures—other drugs have not been studied in this condition, so it is unknown if this is a general class effect

(g) Adverse effects

(1) **All β-blockers have potential to induce bronchospasm** by blocking β_2-receptors; β_1-selective blockers have a lower risk of causing bronchospasm, but the risk is still present

(2) Can precipitate or worsen heart block due to ↓ conduction

(3) Can inhibit insulin release (stimulated by β_1-receptors), worsening glycemic control or inducing frank diabetes in a patient with impaired glucose tolerance

(4) **Can cause dangerous hypoglycemia in diabetics via two mechanisms:** blunting of the normal neurologic response to hypoglycemia so that patients are unaware (e.g., sweating, palpitations, anxiety) and inhibition of glycogenolysis

(5) **Can acutely WORSEN heart failure, and should not be initiated in patients who are fluid-overloaded—** β-blockers should not be started in congestive heart failure until the patient is diuresed to dry weight and other therapies (e.g., ACE inhibitors, digoxin) are at stable doses

3. CNS DRUGS

I. Antipsychotics (see Table 3.1)

A. Typical antipsychotics (neuroleptics/phenothiazines)

    1. Phenothiazines and neuroleptics are synonymous terms for typical antipsychotic agents

    2. Typical antipsychotic agents block dopamine (D) receptors, of which there are five types

    3. Efficacy is proportional to blockade of the type 2 D receptors (D_2 receptors)

    4. Typical agents much more effective at treating positive psychotic symptoms (hallucinations, delusions) than negative symptoms (flat affect, tendency not to speak)

    5. Adverse effects

        (a) **Movement disorders caused by D_2 blockade** (see Table 3.2)

        (b) **Anticholinergic effects** = blurry vision, dry mouth, urinary retention, confusion, loss of memory

        (c) Adrenergic effect = orthostatic hypotension

        (d) **Endocrine effects** = gynecomastia, galactorrhea, amenorrhea ($\uparrow$ prolactin release induced by dopamine blockade)

        (e) Also lower seizure threshold

    6. High versus low potency

        (a) **High potency agents have more D_2 blockade and thus have greater Parkinsonism and less anticholinergic effects**

        (b) **Low potency agents have less D_2 blockade, and thus have less Parkinsonism and more anticholinergic effects**

B. Atypical antipsychotics

    1. **Newer agents, do not work by D_2 antagonism, and efficacy may relate to D_4 or serotonergic receptor antagonism**

    2. Much less marked blockade of D_2 receptors, so these drugs cause **much less extrapyramidal effects** (clozapine causes essentially none)

    3. Due to their superior side effect profile, atypical agents are commonly used 1st line now

Table 3.1 Antipsychotic Agents

Typical Antipsychotics		
Drug	**Potency**	**Characteristics**
haloperidol	High	• Minimal anticholinergic but major movement disorders • Has a depot form for prolonged intramuscular dosing • Useful as a sedative in elderly patients in the ICU, who often respond paradoxically to benzodiazepines • Lowers seizure threshold—avoid in alcohol withdrawal
thiothixene	High	• Minimal anticholinergic but major movement disorders
fluphenazine	High	• Minimal anticholinergic but major movement disorders • Has a depot form for prolonged intramuscular dosing
prochlorperazine	High	• Principally used as an antiemetic
chlorpromazine	Low	• The original phenothiazine, highly sedating
thioridazine	Low	• Minimal movement effects, nonsedating
Atypical Antipsychotics		
Drug	**Characteristics**	
risperidone	• 1st-line agent, fewer movement disorders than any of the typical agents • Higher doses do cause some movement disorders	
olanzapine quetiapine ziprasidone aripiprazole	• 1st-line agents, very minimal movement disorders, generally well tolerated • ziprasidone and aripiprazole cause less weight gain than other atypical agents	
clozapine	• Last-line agent, may work in pts refractory to all other agents • 1% risk of idiosyncratic agranulocytosis, often fatal	

(Continued)

Table 3.1 (Continued)

Atypical Antipsychotics	
Drug	**Characteristics**
	• All pts taking clozapine must have weekly blood draws • Induces NO movement disorders, but has marked anticholinergic effects
Mood Stabilizers	
Drug	**Characteristics**
lithium	• Useful in bipolar syndrome • **Very narrow therapeutic index** • Any cause of renal failure (e.g., ACE inhibitors, dehydration, etc.) → increased lithium-induced toxicity • Toxicities = **nephrogenic diabetes insipidus**, CNS, and thyroid disorders • Major Tx of toxicity is hemodialysis
valproic acid	• Primarily an antiseizure medicine; can be used for bipolar disorder
carbamazepine	• Primarily an antiseizure medicine; can be used for bipolar disorder

C. Mood stabilizers
   1. Lithium
      (a) Mechanism unclear, but stabilizes mood in patients with bipolar syndrome
      (b) Excretion is by the kidneys and is dramatically reduced in patients with renal failure—note that NSAIDs, ACE inhibitors, and dehydration can decrease glomerular filtration, leading to buildup of lithium levels in the blood
      (c) Due to variable pharmacokinetics, blood levels must be periodically monitored
      (d) Adverse effects = tremor, nausea, diarrhea, confusion, ataxia, arrhythmias, polyuria (nephrogenic diabetes insipidus), seizures, hypothyroidism or hyperthyroidism
      (e) **The drug has a very narrow therapeutic window**, meaning that toxicity commonly occurs at therapeutic doses—renal function and thyroid function should be periodically monitored

Table 3.2 Neuroleptic-Induced Movement Disorders

Disorder	Time Course	Characteristics
Acute dystonia	4 hr → 4 days	• Sustained muscle spasm anywhere in the body but often in neck (torticollis), jaw, or back (opisthotonos) • Tx = immediate IV diphenhydramine
Parkinsonism	4 days → 4 mos	• Cog-wheel rigidity, shuffling gait, resting tremor • D_2 blockade upsets the dopamine/acetylcholine balance in the substantia nigra • Tx = benztropine (anticholinergic) to restore balance
Tardive dyskinesia	4 mo → 4 yrs	• Involuntary, irregular movements of the head, tongue, lips, limbs, and trunk • Tx = immediately change medication or ↓ dose • Typically irreversible once sets in
Akathisia	Any time	• Restlessness, pacing, getting up and sitting down • Tx = lower medication doses
Neuroleptic malignant syndrome	Any time	• Life-threatening muscle rigidity → fever, ↑ BP/HR, rhabdomyolysis appearing over 1–3 days • Tx = immediate drug cessation, dantrolene, cool patient, intubate as needed, hydrate with IV fluids

CNS DRUGS

2. Valproic acid & carbamazepine (see section VII)
   (a) Antiseizure medications also indicated as mood stabilizers for bipolar syndrome
   (b) Mechanism unclear

II. Parkinsonian Agents (see Table 3.3)

A. Parkinsonian symptoms are due to an imbalance between dopamine/acetylcholine signaling

B. **Goal of drugs is to ↑ ratio of dopamine to acetylcholine**

C. Can be done by mimicking dopamine signal, increasing dopamine release, inhibiting dopamine metabolism, or inhibiting acetyl-choline signaling

Table 3.3 Parkinsonian Agents

Drug	Characteristics
levodopa (L-dopa)	• Converted to dopamine by dopamine decarboxylase (see Figure 2.3A)
	• 95% of levodopa converted to dopamine in periphery, outside the CNS
	• Because dopamine cannot cross blood-brain barrier, levodopa not efficacious if given by itself, and must be combined with an inhibitor of peripheral dopamine decarboxylase (i.e. carbidopa, see next row)
	• High-protein diet causes competition for levodopa uptake in intestines
levodopa + carbidopa	• First-line therapy for Parkinson's disease, provides marked Sx relief at first
(Sinemet)	• Carbidopa inhibits conversion of dopa to dopamine (see Figure 2.3A)
	• Carbidopa does not cross the blood-brain barrier, so conversion is inhibited in the periphery but occurs in the CNS
	• Adverse effects = nausea, psychosis, anxiety, arrhythmias
	• Chronic use → hyperkinesia/dyskinesias (facial gri-macing, rhythmic jerking movements of hands, head-bobbing, chewing, lip-smacking)
	• May actually speed progression of disease, so some clinicians don't use until late in the disease course
	• Efficacy lost after several years as substantia nigra cells die
	• On-off effect
	⇒ Sudden fluctuations in response can occur over time
	⇒ "On" effect = dyskinesias suddenly develops
	⇒ "Off" effect = akinesia lasting minutes to hours
	• End-of-dose effect = duration of action of each dose shortens

Table 3.3 (Continued)

Drug	Characteristics
entacapone & tolcapone	• Adjunct agents used in combination with levodopa/carbidopa • Inhibit catechol-O-methyltransferase (COMT), so with carbidopa both enzymes that degrade levodopa are inhibited • Results in increased levodopa levels and greater levodopa efficacy, but also increased side effects from the levodopa • Entacapone does not cross BBB but tolcapone does—tolcapone is slightly more effective than entacapone • Beware of drug interactions with other drugs inhibited by COMT enzyme, such as bronchodilators, dopamine agonists, and antihypertensives—can result in neuroleptic malignant syndrome Also, tolcapone linked to case reports of fatal hepatic necrosis
amantadine	• Increases release of dopamine at nerve terminals (see Figure 2.3D) • Less efficacious than Sinemet, most effective in mild disease, and early on • Classic adverse effect = livedo reticularis, a vasculitis effecting the skin, resulting in a lacy appearance of red-blue "fishnet" mottling • Also causes restlessness, hallucinations, dry mouth, urinary retention
bromocriptine pergolide cabergoline ropinirole pramipexole	• Direct agonists of postsynaptic dopamine receptors (see Figure 2.3H) • Often added in patients with inadequate response to Sinemet • Allow reduction in the dose of Sinemet, which can reduce the on-off effect • Also inhibit prolactin secretion (used for prolactinomas) • Have greater incidence of psychiatric complications than levodopa
benztropine trihexyphenidyl biperidin	• Competitively inhibit postsynaptic muscarinic receptors, restoring the dopamine/acetylcholine balance (see Figure 2.2C) • Most effective at treating resting tremor, often in combination with Sinemet

(Continued)

Table 3.3 (Continued)

Drug	Characteristics
	• Adverse effects = sedation, confusion, memory problems, blurry vision, dry mouth, mydriasis, exacerbate glaucoma, arrhythmias, urinary retention • Parkinsonism that is caused by neuroleptics (dopamine antagonists) is often treated with these agents to restore the dopamine/acetylcholine balance
selegiline	• Irreversible inhibitor of MAO_B, prevents dopamine degradation (see Figure 2.3G) • MAO_B is located only in CNS, so selegiline has minimal peripheral effects • Increases efficacy of Sinemet, allowing dose-reduction of Sinemet

III. Stimulants (see Table 3.4)

Table 3.4 CNS Stimulants

Drug	Characteristics
strychnine	• Plant alkaloid, used as a pesticide • Blocks inhibitory CNS glycine receptors → unopposed neuronal signaling • Si/Sx = opisthotonos, severe muscle spasms, convulsions (pseudo-seizures) • Death results from hypoxia • Tx is supportive (e.g., intubation, muscle relaxant)
methylxanthines (caffeine, theophylline)	• Inhibit phosphodiesterase (the enzyme that degrades cAMP) → ↑ cAMP → smooth muscle relaxation • Theophylline used clinically for severe asthmatics, but adverse effects have limited its use more recently • Overall effects of methylxanthines ⇒ ↑ alertness, ↑ HR, ↑ gastric acid production, bronchodilation, diuresis (renal arteriole dilation)

Table 3.4 (Continued)

Drug	Characteristics
	⇒ Dependence is common, leading to withdrawal headaches, and tolerance frequently develops to caffeine
	⇒ Theophylline lowers the seizure threshold
amphetamine	• Indirect sympathomimetic (see Table 2.9)
methylphenidate	• Indirect sympathomimetic (see Table 2.9)
sibutramine	• Indirect sympathomimetic (see Table 2.9)
atomoxetine	• Indirect sympathomimetic (see Table 2.9)
modafinil	• Promotes wakefulness in patients with narcolepsy, sleep apnea, or night shift work
	• Mechanism not clear; side effects include agitation, restlessness, euphoria, alterations in mood
ephedrine	• Mixed sympathomimetic (see Tables 2.8 & 2.9)
cocaine	• Indirect sympathomimetic (see Table 2.9)

IV. Antidepressants (see Table 3.5)

A. Selective serotonin reuptake inhibitors (SSRIs)

   1. **1st line for depression**
   2. Minimal effect on norepinephrine reuptake and minimal muscarinic effects means the side effect profile of SSRIs is superior to tricyclic antidepressants
   3. Few adverse effects, include mild sedation and rare impotence
   4. **SSRIs should not be combined with MAO inhibitors** or serotonin syndrome results
   5. Long half-lives, takes 1–2 mos to wash out of body after termination of Tx

B. Tricyclic antidepressants (TCAs)

   1. 2nd-line agents for depression
   2. Inhibit reuptake of serotonin and norepinephrine at the presynaptic terminus (see Figure 2.3)
   3. Also have anticholinergic properties via blockade of muscarinic receptors, and have some α_1-adrenergic and H_1-receptor blockade

Table 3.5 Antidepressants

Drug	Characteristics
Selective Serotonin Reuptake Inhibitors (SSRIs)	
fluoxetine	• The most stimulatory of the SSRIs, so useful in pts whose depression manifests with negative symptoms (e.g., flat affect, fatigue, etc.)
paroxetine	• The most sedating of the SSRIs, so useful in pts whose depression manifests as anxiety/agitation, and who suffer from severe insomnia
sertraline	• Less stimulatory than fluoxetine, less sedating than paroxetine
citalopram & escitalopram	• Newer SSRIs, escitalopram is the active S enantiomer of citalopram, clinically very similar safety & efficacy
Norepinephrine Stimulators	
duloxetine	• Novel antidepressant works by inhibiting CNS reuptake of serotonin and NE
mirtazapine	• Novel antidepressant works by blocking α_2-receptors, resulting in increased NE release into the synaptic cleft
	• May be associated with rare agranulocytosis
Tricyclic Antidepressants (TCAs)	
amitriptyline	• Tertiary amine, very sedating so should be taken at night
	• Also useful for neuropathic pain, especially diabetic neuropathy
doxepin	• Tertiary amine, very sedating so should be taken at night
imipramine	• Tertiary amine, very sedating so should be taken at night
desipramine	• Secondary amine, less sedating
nortriptyline	• Secondary amine, less sedating
venlafaxine	• A unique drug, actually a "bicyclic" agent, structurally distinct from TCAs
	• Less sedation and orthostatic hypotension than TCAs, but more GI upset

Table 3.5 (Continued)

Drug	Characteristics
Monoamine Oxidase Inhibitors (MAOIs)	
phenelzine tranylcypromine	• Rarely clinically used due to precipitation of serotonin syndrome and hypertensive crisis
Other Agents	
bupropion	• Can lower seizure threshold, but otherwise side effect profile mild

4. Adverse effects = sedation, blurry vision, dry mouth, urinary retention, severe orthostatic hypotension, **QT prolongation → torsade de pointes**
5. Sedating effects mean they are best taken at night
6. Overdoses can cause fatal arrhythmias (QT prolongation) and seizures
7. Divided into tertiary and secondary amines
   (a) Tertiary amines cause more sedation & orthostatic hypotension
   (b) Tertiary amines may thus be useful at night for patients with insomnia

C. Monoamine oxidase inhibitors (MAOIs)

1. 3rd-line agents behind SSRIs and TCAs, very rarely used clinically nowadays
2. Irreversibly inhibit MAO isotypes A & B (unlike selegiline, used for Parkinson's, which only inhibits MAO_B)
3. Because of irreversible inhibition of MAO, before other medicines are started for depression 10–14 days must elapse following discontinuation of MAOIs
4. Severe adverse effects, two classic syndromes
   (a) **Serotonin syndrome**
      (1) Caused by MAOI interaction with SSRI, meperidine, or pseudoephedrine
      (2) Si/Sx = facial flushing, hyperthermia, tachycardia, severe muscle spasm, rhabdomyolysis, altered mental status
      (3) Tx = supportive, cooling agents, muscle relaxants, hydration, intubation if needed

    (b) **Hypertensive crisis**
      (1) Precipitated by ingestion of foods rich in **tyramine**, especially cheese and fermented beverages (e.g., beer, wine), or by sympathomimetic drugs (e.g., ephedrine found in cough or cold medicines)
      (2) Also precipitated by taking TCAs with MAOIs
      (3) Tx = withdrawal of inciting agent and standard BP Tx

D. Bupropion
    1. Mechanism of action not known
    2. Can take several weeks for antidepressant actions to be felt
    3. Also useful to assist with smoking cessation

V. Depressants

A. Benzodiazepines (see Table 3.6)
    1. All have similar anxiolytic properties, but have different pharmacokinetics
      (a) Long half-life drugs include: diazepam (Valium), chlordiazepoxide (Librium)

Table 3.6 Benzodiazepines

Drug	$t_{1/2}$	Characteristics
diazepam	Long	• Metabolized to desmethyldiazepam, an intermediate with a $t_{1/2}$ of 140 hours, so repeated dosing → metabolite buildup • Paradox: **diazepam is very lipophilic so it has very rapid onset of action; however, it rapidly redistributes out of the CNS and into other tissues, so duration of effect following single dose is less than lorazepam, an intermediate-duration drug— after repeated dosing, diazepam builds up in tissues and is no longer redistributed out of the CNS, so its duration of effect is indeed longer than lorazepam** • Commonly used for anxiety, alcohol withdrawal, seizures
chlordiazepoxide	Long	• Also metabolized to desmethyldiazepam • Long half-life makes it suitable for alcohol withdrawal

Table 3.6 (Continued)

Drug	$t_{1/2}$	Characteristics
alprazolam	Mid	• Used as anxiolytic or hypnotic
lorazepam	Mid	• Not metabolized in the liver, useful in pts with liver disease • Widely used as an anxiolytic • **Lorazepam is less lipophilic than diazepam, so lorazepam has a slower onset of action, but a longer duration after a SINGLE dose (it does not redistribute out of the CNS) than diazepam** • Drug of choice in pts with status epilepticus, less commonly used for EtOH withdrawal because of its shorter $t_{1/2}$ after repeat administration
oxazepam	Mid	• Also not metabolized in liver, useful in pts with liver disease
temazepam	Mid	• Used as a hypnotic
midazolam	Short	• Very rapid onset of action, very short half-life • Useful for conscious sedation for procedures, and as a short-acting sedative for radiologic studies (e.g., CT or MRI)
triazolam	Short	• Used as a hypnotic • Because of its short $t_{1/2}$, causes minimal hangover the next morning
Competitive Antagonist		
flumazenil	Short	• Can be used to diagnose benzodiazepine overdose, but is not useful at treating overdose due to its very short $t_{1/2}$, and tendency to induce benzodiazepine withdrawal → seizures

(b) Intermediate half-life drugs include: alprazolam (Xanax), lorazepam (Ativan), oxazepam (Serax), temazepam (Restoril)

(c) Short half-life drugs include: midazolam (Versed), triazolam (Halcion)

2. Bind to the γ-aminobutyric acid (GABA) receptor at a site distinct from the actual GABA binding site (noncompetitive receptor binding)
3. Enhances the effect of GABA binding to the receptor
4. **Highly effective anxiolytics, muscle relaxants, hypnotics, and because of anterograde amnestic properties are often included in anesthesia regimens**
5. **Primary medical use is in alcohol withdrawal, in which benzodiazepines reduce mortality (any benzodiazepine will work for alcohol withdrawal, but longer-acting agents are more commonly used since they are easier to dose)**
6. Hypnotic characteristics
   (a) Hypnotic drugs decrease time to sleep onset (latency period), increase the duration of non–rapid eye movement (NREM) and decrease REM phase sleep, overall increase sleep time
   (b) **Hypnotics do not induce NORMAL sleep**, and therefore the sleep is less restful than normal sleep
   (c) Abrupt cessation can cause withdrawal, leading to REM rebound (increased REM sleep) and nightmares
7. Benzodiazepines have no analgesic properties
8. Adverse effects = confusion (particularly in the elderly), impairment of driving skills, addiction/withdrawal (can be fatal), depression, tolerance
9. Withdrawal effects far more pronounced with short-acting drugs—longer acting drugs have built-in tapering effects
10. Withdrawal Si/Sx = anxiety, insomnia, tremor, seizures (life-threatening)
11. There is cross-tolerance between benzodiazepines, barbiturates, and alcohol
12. **Concurrent administration of alcohol and benzodiazepines is strictly contraindicated—can be fatal**
13. Flumazenil
    (a) A competitive antagonist of benzodiazepine receptors with a very short $t_{1/2}$
    (b) Can precipitate fatal withdrawal seizures in patients on benzodiazepines, so should not be used therapeutically to treat a pt with chronic benzodiazepine use
    (c) Its only real indication is to diagnose benzodiazepine overdose with a one-time dose to see if sedation transiently reverses

B. Barbiturates (see Table 3.7)

1. Like benzodiazepines, barbiturates are divided by pharmacokinetic properties

    (a) Long-acting barbiturate: phenobarbital

    (b) Intermediate-acting barbiturates: secobarbital, pentobarbital

    (c) Ultra-short-acting barbiturates: thiopental, thiamylal

2. The more lipophilic the drug, the faster the rate of entry into the CNS, and thus the faster the onset of action

3. Like benzodiazepines, barbiturates bind to the GABA receptor, potentiating the effects of GABA on the receptor, thereby inhibiting neuronal signaling

4. Metabolism

    (a) Barbiturates are metabolized by hepatic cytochrome p450 enzymes

    (b) **Barbiturates greatly induce the synthesis of p450 enzymes**, especially after chronic barbiturate ingestion

    (c) Thus coumadin, oral contraceptives, digoxin, β-blockers, and other drugs metabolized by p450 have markedly reduced serum levels in pts taking chronic barbiturates

5. Very potent CNS depressants, with a steep dose-response curve

Table 3.7 Barbiturates

Drug	$t_{1/2}$	Characteristics
phenobarbital	Long	• Major clinical use is as a 2nd-line anti-seizure medication
secobarbital, pentobarbital	Mid	• Can be used as powerful sedatives/ hypnotics (sleeping pills)
thiopental, thiamylal	Short	• Rapid onset of action makes them useful as anesthetic agents • After IV administration the drugs are initially distributed to tissues with highest blood flow, especially the brain, inducing rapid anesthesia • The drugs then redistribute to other parts of the body, causing the concentration in the brain to fall, allowing the pt to awaken • Thus termination of anesthesia is due to redistribution, not metabolism

CNS DRUGS

6. **Narrow therapeutic window,** so doses mediating effective sedation and those causing toxic overdose leading to coma and respiratory failure are not far apart

7. Combination with alcohol is especially dangerous, but barbiturates should not be used with benzodiazepines or opiates either

8. **Barbiturates exacerbate acute intermittent porphyria and are therefore absolutely contraindicated in patients with this disease**

9. Tolerance develops over time, and cross-tolerance develops to other sedatives, especially benzodiazepines

10. These drugs are highly addictive

11. Withdrawal can lead to fatal status epilepticus

C. Opioids (narcotics) (see Table 3.8)

1. Opioids are derivatives of opium, which is a poppy-derived mixture of over 20 substances, including morphine and codeine

2. Opioids act via mu (μ), kappa (κ), and delta (δ) receptors to inhibit presynaptic and postsynaptic neurotransmission in the CNS

3. **μ receptors are the dominant receptors at which opioids act to relieve pain**

4. **All opioids cause respiratory depression** (can be fatal), miosis via the parasympathetic Edinger-Westphal nucleus of the 3rd cranial nerve, **nausea/vomiting via direct effect on the chemoreceptor trigger zone** (see Figure 7.2), **cough suppression via direct effect on the cough center in the medulla, severe constipation due to decreased motility and muscle tone in the GI tract,** spasm of the sphincter of Oddi, which may cause a pancreatitis attack, and **histamine release from mast cells causing systemic vasodilation, urticaria, and ↓ BP**

5. **Classic triad of opioid overdose = miosis, respiratory depression, coma**

6. Opioids can be divided into direct agonists, mixed agonist/antagonists, partial agonists, and partial antagonists

   (a) Direct agonists used to treat diarrhea, moderate to severe pain, or cough

   (b) Mixed agonist/antagonists are less addictive and cause less respiratory depression, but may precipitate opioid withdrawal in pts taking other opioids

   (c) Partial agonists and antagonists have less abuse potential, and may be used to treat narcotic overdoses

D. Other agents (see Table 3.9)

Table 3.8 Opioids (Narcotics)

Drug	Characteristics
	Direct Agonists
morphine	• Highly potent opioid, used for relief of severe pain • Variable duration of analgesia—dose to patient's subjective effect, not based on some presumed notion of how long analgesia should last! • Long-acting oral formulations available, or rapid IM/IV administration
codeine	• Less potent than morphine • Used for moderate pain, as antitussive, and for diarrhea • Additive analgesia when combined with acetaminophen or aspirin
oxycodone (Percocet)	• Similar to codeine, typically combined with acetaminophen
hydrocodone (Vicodin)	• Similar to codeine, typically combined with acetaminophen
meperidine (Demerol)	• Much shorter duration of action than morphine, used for severe pain • Causes ↓ spasm of sphincter of Oddi, so may be preferred for pancreatitis • Lowers seizure threshold! • Absolute contraindication in pts taking MAOIs to prevent serotonin syndrome
fentanyl	• Most potent opioid (80× more potent than morphine), used for severe pain • Very rapid acting and rapid wear-off, useful for anesthesia for bedside procedures and for electrical cardioversion • Comes in a patch for chronic pain relief in pts who can't take orals
diphenoxylate (Lomotil)	• Used to treat diarrhea, limited CNS effects • Not useful for pain relief
loperamide	• Used to treat diarrhea, limited CNS effects • Not useful for pain relief

(Continued)

CNS DRUGS

Table 3.8 (Continued)

Drug	Characteristics
methadone	• Long duration of action, most useful to treat heroin addiction because withdrawal from methadone is much milder
dextromethorphan	• No analgesic activity, but potent antitussive activity • Principally found in over-the-counter antitussive medications
propoxyphene (Darvon)	• Relatively weak analgesic, may be used for mild to moderate pain • Better efficacy if combined with acetaminophen or aspirin
Mixed Agonist/Antagonists	
pentazocine (Darvon)	• Less potency and efficacy than morphine for pain relief • Less addictive and less respiratory depression than morphine • May cause cardiovascular stimulation at high doses, avoid in coronary disease
nalbuphine	• Similar to pentazocine, but does not cause cardiovascular stimulation
butorphanol	• Similar to pentazocine, but its potency is similar to morphine
Partial Agonists & Antagonists	
buprenorphine	• Partial agonist, more potent than morphine due to slow receptor dissociation • May be used as an alternative to methadone for heroin detoxification
naloxone (Narcan)	• Partial antagonist used to treat opioid overdose • Must be given parenterally, has a short $t_{1/2}$, so repeated doses are required
naltrexone	• Similar to naloxone, but can be given orally and is longer acting

Table 3.9 CNS Depressants: Other Agents

Drug	Characteristics
buspirone	• Totally distinct mechanism, serotonin agonist ($5HT_{1A}$ receptor) • Used as an anxiolytic, but causes minimal sedation, takes 3–8 weeks for effect • Lacks antiseizure and muscle relaxant properties of benzodiazepines • Few adverse effects, primarily headache, minimal tolerance, & withdrawal • No dangerous interaction with alcohol, but abruptly switching patients from benzodiazepines to buspirone can induce benzodiazepine withdrawal
propranolol	• Because it is so lipophilic, it crosses the blood-brain barrier • 1st-line indication for performance anxiety, also useful for central tremors
zolpidem eszopiclone	• Interact with the GABA receptor, although the drugs are not benzodiazepines • Used as sedative-hypnotics for insomnia
ethanol (alcohol)	• Used as topical disinfectant & given IV for methanol & ethylene glycol ingestion • Rapidly absorbed from the GI tract by passive diffusion, but food delays uptake • Alcohol dehydrogenase converts ethanol to acetaldehyde, a toxic intermediate that is normally rapidly broken down to acetate by aldehyde dehydrogenase • Disulfiram inhibits aldehyde dehydrogenase → acetaldehyde buildup → terrible headaches, vomiting, chest pain, can be dangerous and not an effective treatment for alcoholism so rarely used nowadays • Some ethnic groups, especially Asians, have an aldehyde dehydrogenase isoenzyme that does not quickly convert acetaldehyde to acetate, so alcohol causes vasodilation, facial flushing, tachycardia, and headache in these people • Cytochrome p450 ⇒ Acute intake of alcohol occupies p450 enzymes, competitively antagonizing metabolism of other p450-dependent drugs → ↑ serum levels of those drugs

CNS DRUGS

(Continued)

Table 3.9 (Continued)

Drug	Characteristics
	⇒ Chronic intake of alcohol massively induces p450 enzyme synthesis → ↑ metabolism of p450-dependent drugs → ↓ serum levels of those drugs
	• CNS depression
	⇒ Effects not mediated by a specific alcohol receptor
	⇒ Ethanol dissolves in neuronal cell membranes, disrupting normal function
	⇒ Early → euphoria, behavior activation/disinhibition (↑ talking, ↑ aggression)
	⇒ Later → relaxation, anxiolytic, slurred speech, impaired judgment, sleep
	⇒ Higher doses cause respiratory failure, coma, and then death
	• Other organ system effects
	⇒ Peripheral vasodilation (direct effect) → hypothermia
	⇒ Depression of myocardial contractility → dilated cardiomyopathy over time
	⇒ Gastritis, GI bleeding, pancreatitis, fatty liver, hepatitis → fibrosis over time
	⇒ Peripheral neuropathy & Wernicke-Korsakoff syndrome (confabulation, ataxia, ophthalmoplegia)
	• Withdrawal
	⇒ 4 syndromes: tremor, seizure, hallucinations, delirium tremens (DTs)
	⇒ Seizures and DTs (autonomic instability) are potentially fatal
	⇒ All manifestations treated with benzodiazepines

VI. Muscle Relaxants (see Table 3.10)

VII. Antiseizure Drugs

A. Monotherapy is preferred and is successful in most cases

B. Some patients require multidrug therapy, but be careful of drug interactions in these patients

C. Drug therapy depends on the nature of the seizures (see Table 3.11)

D. Different drugs can be used in more than one type of seizure (see Table 3.12)

Table 3.10 Muscle Relaxants

Drug	Characteristics
baclofen	• GABA analog, works in spinal cord • Useful as a general muscle relaxant and in patients with low back pain
cyclobenzaprine	• Works at the level of the brain stem and is structurally related to tricyclic antidepressants • Not recommended in cerebral palsy, patients on MAOIs, or with arrhythmias
dantrolene	• Works peripherally as a skeletal muscle relaxant • Inhibits calcium release from sarcoplasmic reticulum, blocking skeletal muscle contraction • 1st line for neuroleptic malignant syndrome and malignant hypertension
diazepam	• GABA-ergic enhancer, useful for serious muscle spasms
tizanidine	• Central-acting α_2 agonist similar to clonidine • Acts as an antispasmodic agent for patients with muscle spasticity from multiple sclerosis and spinal cord injury
Botox	• Botulinum toxin, blocks neuromuscular transmission by blocking cleavage of SNAP-25 on the presynaptic nerve terminal, inhibiting the release of acetylcholine • Used to treat cervical dystonia, axillary hyperhidrosis (↑ sweating), strabismus, blepharospasm

Table 3.11 Antiseizure Medications by Seizure Type

Generalized Seizures	
Absence (petit mal)	
◆ Brief period of unresponsiveness (<30 seconds), pt stares blankly	
1st line	• ethosuximide, valproic acid
2nd line	• lamotrigine
Tonic-Clonic (grand mal)	
◆ Dramatic convulsions with loss of consciousness, incontinence, postictal confusion	
1st line	• valproic acid, carbamazepine, phenytoin
2nd line	• lamotrigine, phenobarbital, primidone

(Continued)

Table 3.11 (Continued)

Generalized Seizures

Partial Seizures

Simple Partial	
◆ Sensory seizure or limited, focal motor seizure	
1st line	• carbamazepine, phenytoin, levetiracetam
2nd line	• gabapentin, lamotrigine, phenobarbital, primidone, topiramate, valproic acid

Complex Partial	
◆ Starts as simple partial but then generalizes	
1st line	• carbamazepine, phenytoin, levetiracetam
2nd line	• gabapentin, lamotrigine, phenobarbital, primidone, topiramate, valproic acid

Status Epilepticus	
◆ Unremitting seizure → respiratory compromise & rhabdomyolysis	
1st line	• lorazepam, diazepam
2nd line	• phenytoin
3rd line	• phenobarbital coma

Table 3.12 Antiseizure Medications

Drug	Seizure Type	Characteristics
ethosuximide	• Absence (1st line)	• Nonsedating, causes mild GI side effects, rare idiosyncratic blood dyscrasias
valproic acid	• Absence (1st line) • Tonic-clonic (1st line) • Partial (2nd line)	• Can cause hepatotoxicity, blood dyscrasias • Also useful for bipolar syndrome
phenytoin	• Tonic-clonic (1st line) • Partial (1st line) • Status epilepticus (2nd line)	• Nonsedating, causes gingival hyperplasia, hirsutism, hypotension during IV load • Major inducer of cytochrome p450 enzymes • Can cause hepatic toxicity in patients with underlying liver disease

Table 3.12 (Continued)

Drug	Seizure Type	Characteristics
carbamazepine	• Partial (1st line) • Tonic-clonic (1st line)	• Causes blood dyscrasias, headaches, rashes • Also used to treat trigeminal neuralgia & bipolar syndrome • Contraindicated in absence seizures
levetiracetam	• Partial (1st line)	• Mechanism unknown • Very well tolerated
tiagabine	• Partial (adjunctive)	• Enhances GABA signaling
zonisamide	• Partial (adjunctive)	• Unique mechanism, blocks sodium and calcium channels • Kidney stones may occur
phenobarbital	• Partial (2nd line) • Tonic-clonic (2nd line) • Status epilepticus (3rd line)	• Stimulates GABA signaling • Highly sedating, addictive • Marked cytochrome p450 enzyme induction • 3rd line for status by putting pt into a coma
primidone	• Partial (3rd line) • Tonic-clonic (3rd line)	• Metabolized to phenobarbital • Poorly tolerated, seldom used
gabapentin	• Partial (2nd line) • Tonic-clonic (2nd line)	• A GABA analog • An adjunctive therapy, not used by itself • Minor side effects include dizziness, ataxia • Also useful for neuropathic pain syndromes • Few drug interactions, ideal as adjunctive Tx
lamotrigine	• Partial (2nd line)	• May inhibit release of glutamate in the brain

(*Continued*)

Table 3.12 (Continued)

Drug	Seizure Type	Characteristics
		• Used as adjunct therapy, not by itself • Markedly alters levels of other antiepileptics • Causes headache, GI upset, rash
felbamate	• Partial (3rd line)	• Mechanism unclear, may relate to GABA • Used as monotherapy or adjunctive therapy • Blood dyscrasias & hepatotoxicity can be severe; reserve for refractory patients
topiramate	• Partial (2nd line) • Tonic-clonic (2nd line)	• Mechanism unclear, may relate to GABA • Causes cognitive slowing, tremor, GI upset • Used as adjunctive therapy in refractory pts
diazepam	• Status epilepticus (1st line) • Alcohol withdrawal seizure (1st line)	• Onset is faster than lorazepam, but remember, redistribution of diazepam means that with a one-time dose its duration is shorter than lorazepam
lorazepam	• Status epilepticus (1st line) • Alcohol withdrawal seizure (1st line)	• Onset is slower than diazepam, but because of slower redistribution, with a one-time dose lorazepam effect lasts longer than diazepam

VIII. Neuroprotective Agents

A. Memantine
1. Novel Alzheimer's drug
2. An N-methyl-D-aspartate (NMDA) receptor antagonist that reduces glutamatergic excitotoxicity, preventing apoptosis of neurons
3. May have efficacy in other forms of dementia as well
B. Riluzole
1. Slows progression of amyotrophic lateral sclerosis (ALS)
2. Exact mechanism unclear, but may involve inhibition of glutamate toxicity to nerves

IX. Drugs of Abuse (see Table 3.13)

A. Opioids (e.g., heroin)
1. Rush obtained after opiate injection is directly proportional to the lipophilicity of the agent
2. Severity of withdrawal is inversely proportional to half-life
B. Cocaine
1. Three phases of withdrawal
(a) 1st phase (the "crash")
(1) First phase, patient feels irritable, confused, dysphoric, possibly suicidal
(2) Insomnia despite physical exhaustion
(3) Finally sleep for 8–40 hrs and wake up extremely hungry
(b) 2nd phase
(1) Lasts from 2–10 weeks
(2) Sleep patterns normalize, mood improves
(3) Late in 2nd phase anxiety and irritability develop, anhedonia develops, leading to a return for the craving for cocaine
(c) 3rd phase
(1) Baseline mood reestablished but with episodic cocaine cravings
(2) Environmental cues (e.g., cocaine-using friends, seeing sugar spilled on the table) trigger the cravings
2. **Cocaine acts at the presynaptic dopamine terminal, blocking reuptake of dopamine and other catecholamines** (see Figure 2.3F)

Table 3.13 Drugs of Abuse

Drug	Characteristics
heroin	• Highly lipophilic → rapid rush, short half-life = 3–5 hrs • Combined with cocaine in "speed-balls" • Withdrawal begins 4–6 hrs after last dose, peaks at 48 hrs, subsides in 7–10 days • Treatment – Addiction → methadone – Overdose → naloxone or naltrexone – Withdrawal → clonidine
cocaine	• Increased catecholamine signaling at the neurosynaptic junction leads to acute coronary vasospasm & cerebral vasospasm → myocardial infarction, arrhythmias, stroke, intracranial bleeds, aortic dissection • Cocaine also causes early-onset atherosclerosis
amphetamine	• Causes tremor, mydriasis, hypertension, hyperthermia, ↑ myocardial demand → myocardial infarction or stroke/intracranial bleed • Can also cause acute psychosis and violence
MDMA	• Causes visual and other sensory hallucinations • Pts feel increased perceptions of self-insight, heightened empathy with others • Causes neurotoxicity that can be indistinguishable from Parkinson's disease
PCP	• Causes psychosis, hallucinations, panic, violence, can mimic schizophrenia • Pts unaware of pain so can perform amazing feats, such as breaking out of hard restraints while breaking a limb-bone or dislocating a limb without noticing it
marijuana	• Causes euphoria and relaxation, alteration of time perception, decreased cognition, reduction in short-term memory, dose-dependent tachycardia, and classic conjunctival injection • Inhalation, like cigarettes, increases risk of bronchitis, asthma, and squamous cell metaplasia
LSD	• Causes classic sense inversion: the pt sees sounds, hears colors, smells sights, etc. • Hallucinations consist of vivid colors in kaleidoscopes
mescaline	• Similar to LSD

C. Amphetamine
   1. Causes ↑ energy, self-confidence, loss of appetite, euphoria
   2. Acts at the presynaptic nerve terminus, causing release of biological amines (see Figure 2.3D)

D. MDMA (methylene dioxymethamphetamine, "ecstasy")
   1. Causes serotonin release and blocks reuptake of serotonin
   2. Also increases extracellular dopamine and norepinephrine

E. Phencyclidine (PCP, angel dust)
   1. Related to ketamine, causes a sensation of a person being removed from their body, or floating
   2. Has potent analgesic properties

F. Marijuana
   1. Derived from the hemp plant, its active compounds are cannabinoids
   2. Tetrahydrocannabinol is the primary psychoactive agent

G. LSD (lysergic acid diethylamide)
   1. An ergot alkaloid derivative, agonist/antagonist of serotonin receptors

H. Mescaline
   1. Also a hallucinogenic alkaloid, used by Native Americans in some religious ceremonies

I. Acamprosate
   1. Mechanism relates to GABA receptor agonism, although not entirely understood
   2. Increases rate of abstinence in alcoholics trying to stay sober

J. Rimonabant
   1. Developmental agent in phase III clinical trials as an appetite suppressant for obesity and diabetes; may also help with smoking cessation
   2. Works by the novel mechanism of blocking the cannaboid receptor

4. ANTI-INFLAMMATORY AGENTS

I. Acetaminophen (see Table 4.1)

A. **Potent analgesic and antipyretic activity but has** anti-inflammatory activity

B. **Far superior side effect and safety profile versus nonsteroidal anti-inflammatory (NSAID) agents,** causing no gastritis/ulcers, no worsening of bleeding diathesis, no impairment of glomerular filtration rate, and no Reye's syndrome in children with chicken pox or influenza

C. Mechanism of action remains a mystery

D. 1st-line analgesic for run-of-the-mill pain

E. The drug is a weak base, with a high pK_a, and is absorbed in the small intestine

F. **Toxic overdoses can cause fatal hepatic necrosis and renal failure,** but the drug has a large therapeutic index, and therapeutic doses are typically much lower than toxic doses

G. **Drug overdose is easily treated, if started early, with N-acetylcysteine,** an antioxidant that helps metabolize the toxic intermediate of acetaminophen formed in the liver

II. Aspirin (Acetylsalicylic Acid)

A. An excellent analgesic, anti-inflammatory, antipyretic, and antiplatelet agent

B. **Irreversibly inhibits cyclooxygenase** (isoforms 1 and 2), preventing prostaglandin and thromboxane formation (see Figure 6.1)

C. Toxicity

    1. Aspirin is an organic acid, which can cause direct toxicity to the gastric mucosa, leading to gastritis and ulcer formation

    2. Aspirin irreversibly acetylates platelets and can cause bleeding in patients predisposed to bleeding

    3. For unclear reasons, the use of aspirin in children with febrile viral infections (e.g., chicken pox) is associated with Reye's syndrome, a fatal, fulminant hepatic failure

    4. Aspirin can exacerbate gout because it inhibits renal tubular secretion of uric acid

Table 4.1 Anti-Inflammatory Agents

Drug	Characteristics
acetaminophen	• 1st-line agent for mild to moderate pain, excellent safety profile • Remember, although often considered an NSAID, acetaminophen does not have anti-inflammatory activity; it is strictly an analgesic
aspirin	• 1st line to prevent coronary syndromes—proven to ↓ mortality in pts at risk for coronary dz, & to ↓ mortality acutely in ischemic pts • 1st line to prevent stroke in patients at risk • 2nd line for patients with atrial fibrillation (behind Coumadin) • Can be used, cautiously, for minor aches and pains, but should not be used in patients with bleeding diatheses or ulcers, or gout
NSAIDs (e.g., ibuprofen, naproxen, etc.)	• Can be used for mild to moderate pain of a variety of causes • Unlike aspirin, these are 1st-line agents for gout • Avoid in pts with congestive heart failure (can worsen renal function) • Be careful in patients with wounds or bleeding diatheses
COX-2 inhibitors	• Celecoxib available, rofecoxib and valdecoxib withdrawn from the market • Selective inhibition of COX-2 spares COX-1 inhibition in GI mucosa, resulting in diminished risk of GI bleeding • However, increased risk of cardiovascular events, including myocardial infarctions, may result from unopposed thromboxane activation via COX-1
antimalarials	• Particularly useful for skin manifestations of collagen vascular diseases • Allow reduction in steroid doses, major side effect is chorioretinitis
gold salts	• Seldom used, because of hepatic/renal/blood toxicities

(Continued)

Table 4.1 (Continued)

Drug	Characteristics
penicillamine	• Seldom used, because of renal/blood toxicity
thalidomide	• Blocks TNF secretion, improves healing of skin ulcers, and improves outcome in leprosy & multiple myeloma • Infamous teratogen
pentoxifylline	• Blocks TNF secretion, improves survival in alcoholic hepatitis
infliximab	• Monoclonal anti-TNF antibody, used in rheumatoid arthritis & Crohn's dz
adalimumab	• Humanized anti-TNF monoclonal antibody similar to infliximab
etanercept	• Recombinant TNF receptor, used in rheumatoid arthritis
anakinra	• Recombinant human interleukin-1 receptor antagonist • Akin to TNF blockers, this drug blocks the effect of interleukin-1 in rheumatoid arthritis—used as an adjunct agent with other drugs
leflunomide	• Antimetabolite, inhibits leukocyte replication, used for rheumatoid arthritis
efalizumab	• Anti-CD11a monoclonal antibody prevents leukocyte influx into psoriatic skin
colchicine	• Used for gout—lower therapeutic index than NSAIDs
uricosuric agents	• Probenecid and sulfinpyrazone, useful for chronic gout • Remember, can precipitate an acute gout flare when first started
allopurinol	• Used for overproducers of uric acid for chronic gout therapy
azathioprine	• Used for refractory rheumatoid arthritis, maintenance of solid organ transplants, inflammatory bowel disease, and in other autoimmune dz • Allopurinol antagonizes the effect of azathioprine by inhibiting its conversion to its active metabolite, mercaptopurine

Table 4.1 (Continued)

Drug	Characteristics
methotrexate	• Used for rheumatoid arthritis, psoriasis, chemotherapy • Over 1 gram total dose increases the risk of hepatic fibrosis
mesalamine/ sulfasalazine	• Pro-drugs converted to their active drug, 5-aminosalicylate, by colonic bacteria, used for inflammatory bowel disease
mycophenolate	• Inhibits lymphocyte proliferation, useful for solid organ transplants
rapamycin	• Inhibits lymphocyte activation, useful for solid organ transplants
antithymocyte globulin	• Kills T cells, used rarely now for autoimmune disorders
OKT3	• A monoclonal antibody that kills T cells, useful during acute rejection of solid organ transplants
cyclosporine	• Inhibits T-cell proliferation, useful for solid organ transplants
FK-506	• Inhibits T-cell proliferation, useful for solid organ transplants
glucocorticoids	• See Endocrine, section III
basiliximab	• Anti-CD25 antibody (anti-IL-2-receptor α chain)
daclizumab	• Blocks lymphocyte activation/proliferation, used to prevent solid organ graft rejection
glatiramer	• An amino acid polymer based on myelin structure that induces T-suppressor cells and ameliorates multiple sclerosis
omalizumab	• Anti-IgE monoclonal antibody for refractory asthma

5. **Aspirin overdose causes a classic syndrome**
   (a) **Tinnitus, fever, and acute respiratory alkalosis are the classic triad of acute overdose**
   (b) Eventually metabolic collapse ensues, and a metabolic acidosis overwhelms the alkalosis
   (c) Because aspirin is a weak organic acid, it is absorbed in the stomach (protonated in the low pH environment, neutralizing its own charge, allowing it to cross biological membranes)

      (d) Gastric lavage and activated charcoal should immediately be administered to prevent additional gastric absorption

      (e) **Alkalinization of the urine causes ion trapping of aspirin by deprotonating it in the renal tubules,** thereby giving it a negative charge and preventing it from crossing back into the peritubular capillaries

III. Nonsteroidal Anti-Inflammatory Drugs (NSAIDs)

A. There are dozens available now; for the most part they can be divided into nonselective and selective NSAIDs

B. Nonselective NSAIDs reversibly inhibit cyclooxygenase isoforms 1 and 2 (COX-1, COX-2) (see Figure 6.1)

C. Selective NSAIDs reversibly inhibit COX-2 much more potently than COX-1

D. COX-1 inhibition is responsible for the majority of the gastritis and ulcer formation associated with standard NSAIDs

E. COX-2 is the dominant isoform active during inflammation (although COX-1 also plays a role)

F. Selective inhibition of COX-2 is therefore less likely to cause GI bleeding than nonselective inhibitors; **however, it is now known that COX-2 inhibitors increase the risk of myocardial infarction probably via increased exposure to pro-thrombotic thromboxane due to unopposed COX-1 activity**

G. **Other adverse effects of NSAIDs include reduction of glomerular filtration rate in patients with congestive heart failure** (due to their dependence on prostaglandin E to dilate preglomerular arterioles to maintain perfusion pressure to the glomeruli), and reversible acetylation of platelets leading to increased bleeding from cuts and wounds—neither of these adverse effects are diminished in selective COX-2 inhibitors

H. Aspirin can inhibit uric acid secretion in the renal tubules, and should NOT be used to treat gout

IV. Agents for Autoimmune Diseases

A. Antimalarial drugs

    1. These drugs are quinine derivatives: chloroquine, hydroxychloroquine, quinacrine

    2. Their anti-inflammatory mechanism of action is not known, but they are effective for a variety of collagen vascular diseases, including systemic lupus erythematosus and rheumatoid arthritis

B. Gold salts
   1. Mechanism of action unknown, but can be useful for refractory rheumatoid arthritis
   2. Cause severe skin rash, hepatic/renal damage, blood dyscrasias—seldom used anymore

C. Penicillamine
   1. Mechanism of action unknown, but can be useful for refractory rheumatoid arthritis
   2. Causes renal toxicity and blood dyscrasia—seldom used
   3. Is used as a copper chelator in Wilson's disease

D. Leflunomide
   1. Inhibits leukocyte replication by inhibiting dihydroorotate dehydrogenase, thereby blocking RNA and DNA synthesis
   2. Used for rheumatoid arthritis
   3. Major side effects are hepatotoxicity and cytopenias

E. Anti–tumor necrosis factor (TNF) therapy
   1. TNF is a key regulator of inflammation and acts in a variety of disease states
   2. Five drugs currently available to reduce TNF levels
      (a) Thalidomide
         (1) Thalidomide inhibits secretion and peripheral effects of TNF
         (2) **It causes severe birth defects and must not be used in menstruating women unless they agree a priori to take birth control,** and even then with caution!
         (3) It has been proven useful in therapy for leprosy, chronic skin ulcers (e.g., pyoderma gangrenosa), HIV-associated mucosal ulcers, and for multiple myeloma
      (b) Pentoxifylline
         (1) A phosphodiesterase inhibitor that inhibits TNF (and other cytokine) secretion
         (2) Also inhibits platelet aggregation, and therefore has been used as an aspirin-like anticoagulant in patients with peripheral vascular disease
         (3) Improves survival in acute alcoholic hepatitis
      (c) Infliximab (anti-TNF monoclonal antibody)
         (1) A humanized, murine monoclonal antibody directed against TNF

(2) Neutralizes TNF and can be given IV once per 4–8 weeks because of a prolonged serum half-life ($t_{1/2}$ of IgG in the body is 2–4 weeks)

(3) Shown very promising results in patients with rheumatoid arthritis and in Crohn's disease, allowing steroid doses to be tapered down with dramatic symptom relief

(4) Major side effects are rare transfusion reactions and delayed serum sickness

(5) **Its use has been associated with the development of sudden sepsis and disseminated mycobacterial disease in some patients**

(d) Adalimumab

(1) Humanized anti-TNF monoclonal antibody similar to infliximab

(2) Dosed SQ instead of IV

(e) Etanercept (recombinant TNF receptor)

(1) A chimeric protein (made of different parts fused together) composed of the recombinant receptor for TNF and the constant region of an immunoglobulin

(2) Neutralizes TNF in the bloodstream

(3) Shown very promising results in patients with rheumatoid arthritis, allowing steroid doses to be tapered down with dramatic symptom relief

(4) Administered subcutaneously every week

(5) Few side effects, mostly local injection reactions

(6) Like infliximab, **etanercept has been associated with the development of sudden sepsis and with disseminated mycobacterial infections**

F. Anakinra

1. Recombinant human interleukin-1 receptor antagonist—blocks activity of interleukin-1 in inflamed joints in rheumatoid arthritis

2. Improves signs and symptoms of moderate to severe rheumatoid arthritis

3. May increase susceptibility to infections

G. Efalizumab

1. Anti-CD11a monoclonal antibody blocks integrin-mediated translocation of leukocytes from blood vessels into inflamed, psoriatic skin

2. Predominant side effect is infusion reaction, but may also increase risk of infections

H. Omalizumab: an anti-IgE monoclonal antibody used for patients with asthma refractory to standard therapy

V. Drugs for Uric Acid and/or Gout

A. **NSAIDs are 1st-line agents for gout, but aspirin should be avoided because of its potential to inhibit uric acid secretion from the renal tubules**

B. Colchicine
    1. Can be used prophylactically or therapeutically for acute attack
    2. Works by preventing microtubular function, thereby preventing discharge of inflammatory granules by leukocytes
    3. At high doses it poisons rapidly dividing cells, such as white blood cells, but also GI tract lining cells
    4. Can cause GI ulceration, diarrhea, and agranulocytosis
    5. Less commonly used now due to its potential toxicity

C. Probenecid & sulfinpyrazone
    1. **Uricosuric agents**—promote the renal excretion of uric acid by preventing tubular reabsorption of urea
    2. Should only be used if an anti-inflammatory agent is being taken (e.g., colchicine or NSAID), because they **can cause an acute flair of gout when first started**
    3. Lowering uric acid levels over the long term prevents tissue deposition

D. Allopurinol
    1. Inhibits xanthine oxidase, the rate-limiting step in purine catabolism
    2. This prevents formation of uric acid, thus lowering uric acid levels over time
    3. Most useful in patients who "overproduce" uric acid as a cause of their gout, as opposed to "underexcreters" who may benefit more from uricosuric agents

E. Rasburicase
    1. Recombinant urate oxidase; breaks apart uric acid
    2. Used for severe hyperuricemia associated with tumor lysis syndrome
    3. Predominant adverse effect is anaphylaxis; the drug can also cause hemolysis in G6PDH deficient patients because as it splits uric acid a byproduct is formation of hydrogen peroxide, which soaks up reducing agents (e.g., NADPH)

VI. Immunosuppressives

A. Antimetabolites

1. Azathioprine

(a) A precursor of 6-mercaptopurine, and hence, a purine analog

(b) **Xanthine oxidase converts azathioprine to mercaptopurine, so the effects of azathioprine depend on functional xanthine oxidase—never mix allopurinol and azathioprine together in the same patient!**

(c) Conversion to mercaptopurine inhibits synthesis of new nucleotides in rapidly dividing cells, principally white blood cells

(d) Azathioprine has a variety of indications for immunosuppression

2. Methotrexate

(a) **Inhibits dihydrofolate reductase**, an enzyme necessary for nucleotide synthesis in rapidly dividing cells

(b) **Causes a dose-related hepatic fibrosis** as well as GI and bone marrow toxicity, both of which are diminished by co-administration of folinic acid, which acts downstream of the block methotrexate mediates in the folate pathway

(c) Useful for a variety of immunosuppressive, chemotherapeutic, and dermatologic disorders

3. Mesalamine/sulfasalazine

(a) Mesalamine is 5-aminosalicylate, which can be administered rectally for inflammatory bowel disease

(b) **Sulfasalazine is a conjugated molecule that is poorly absorbed from the intestine and that colonic bacteria split into two components, sulfapyridine (a carrier molecule) and 5-aminosalicylate, the latter of which mediates the anti-inflammatory effects**

4. Mycophenolate mofetil

(a) Inhibits the de novo synthetic pathway of purines

(b) Powerful inhibitor of lymphocyte proliferation

(c) Favorable side effect profile has led to its use as a 1st-line immunosuppressive for solid organ transplants, sparing the use of the more toxic cyclosporine

5. Rapamycin

(a) A derivative of macrolide antibiotics; inhibits the response of leukocytes to stimulatory signals

(b) Also used for organ transplantation

B. Antilymphocyte therapies
   1. Antithymocyte globulin (ATG)
      (a) Polyclonal antibody obtained by immunizing horses with human T lymphocytes
      (b) Very potently and nonspecifically shuts down or kills T cells, but effects can last for years after dosing
      (c) Rarely used now, but still occasionally used in aplastic anemia or other autoimmune blood disorders
   2. Antilymphocyte monoclonal antibodies (see Table 4.1)
   3. Cyclosporine
      (a) Inhibits calcineurin, and calcineurin turns on the interleukin-2 (IL-2) gene, and IL-2 is required for T cell proliferation, so **cyclosporine suppresses T cell proliferation**
      (b) Revolutionized solid organ transplant, but toxicities are not benign
      (c) It is directly nephrotoxic, causes hypertension, hypercholesterolemia, and possibly early atherosclerosis
   4. FK-506
      (a) Like cyclosporine, it inhibits calcineurin, and thereby inhibits IL-2 secretion and T-cell proliferation
      (b) It is more potent than cyclosporine but has similar toxicities
      (c) It is also used in solid organ transplants
C. Glucocorticoids (see Endocrine, section III)

5. ANESTHETICS

I. Local Anesthetics

A. General principles

1. **All local anesthetics have three components**

    (a) Lipophilic aromatic ring

    (b) Intermediate connecting chain with either an ester or amide

        (1) Ester anesthetics are rapidly hydrolyzed by plasma cholinesterases

        (2) Some people are "slow acetylators," meaning they have unusually slow cholinesterases, and the effects of these drugs last an unusually long time

        (3) Amide anesthetics are metabolized in the liver, and toxicity can occur in pts with liver dz

    (c) Hydrophilic amine at the other end with an ionizable side group

2. Local anesthetics come as salts in solution

3. pK_a typically 8 to 9 (weak bases), so at physiologic pH the ionized form dominates

4. Toxicity depends on systemic absorption, and rate of absorption depends on the dose given, the blood flow to the area administered, and physiochemical properties of the drug

5. The ionized form is the active form because it binds to the receptor site, which is on the cytoplasmic face of the cell membrane

6. **However, the un-ionized form is crucial because it is much better able to diffuse through the cell membrane to reach the active site—in areas of inflammation, local tissue pH drops, ionizing the anesthetics extracellularly, thereby preventing their crossing into cells to mediate an anesthetic effect**

7. **Vasoconstrictor (often epinephrine) is often added to topical anesthetics to limit absorption by decreasing blood flow to the area**, which prevents bleeding in the surgical field—addition of 1% epinephrine to lidocaine increases the toxic dose from 4 mg/kg to 7 mg/kg (almost double)

8. Mechanism of all local anesthetics is stabilization of cell membrane, preventing depolarization of peripheral nerves

Table 5.1 Local Anesthetics

Drug	Amide/Ester	Characteristics
benzocaine	Ester	• Only topical use, poorly absorbed, no systemic toxicity
cocaine	Ester	• Only topical use, excellent absorption → systemic toxicity • Unique local agent in that it causes vasoconstriction by itself
chloroprocaine	Ester	• Used in obstetrics (rapidly hydrolyzed, no effects on fetus)
lidocaine	Amide	• Most commonly used local agent, used for all types of locals
bupivacaine	Amide	• Prolonged duration of action

ANESTHETICS

9. Nerve fibers with smaller diameters are affected first—autonomic fibers blocked first, then pain fibers, then motor fibers

10. Types of local anesthesia
    (a) Topical—affecting mucous membranes
    (b) Infiltration—injection under skin
    (c) Regional blocks
        (1) Spinal anesthesia is injection into the cerebrospinal fluid (CSF) to block signaling in the cord past the area of injection
        (2) Lumbar epidural anesthesia is injection outside the dura, allows localization of effect to a specific spinal segment, bordered on both sides by unaffected areas
        (3) Caudal anesthesia is drug injection through the sacral hiatus above the coccyx

B. Drugs (see Table 5.1)

II. General Anesthetics

A. General principles

1. Anesthetic drugs do not elicit their pharmacological actions by interacting with selective receptors, but instead affect cell membrane fluid dynamics

2. **The potency of anesthetics correlates with their oil/water partition coefficient,** because more hydrophobic agents diffuse more readily into the plasma membranes in the CNS

3. Unconsciousness is produced when a specific concentration of anesthetic agent is achieved in CNS cell membranes

4. Inhalational anesthetics are inert gases that interact with tissues and liquids physically as gases rather than chemically in solution

5. Henry's law
   (a) Volume of gas in liquid = partial pressure in solution × solubility
   (b) When anesthetic agents are administered, a partial pressure equilibrium is achieved between the undissolved and dissolved gas in the liquid, such that the agent is transported in the blood as an equilibrium mixture of soluble and gaseous forms
   (c) The effects of an agent are only mediated when the partial pressure of the gas achieves some minimal threshold in biological membranes
   (d) Henry's law tells us that at a constant volume, a lower solubility causes an inversely proportionate increase in partial pressure, so **agents that have LOWER water solubility tend to have HIGHER anesthetic potency** (meaning they induce anesthesia at lower concentrations in the serum)

6. Minimum alveolar concentration (MAC)
   (a) **MAC ≡ the concentration of drug that results in immobility in 50% of patients** when exposed to a standardized surgical skin incision
   (b) Units of MAC = % inhaled gas at 1 atmosphere
   (c) MAC is thus a measure of potency—**low MAC indicates low water solubility and high potency**
   (d) MAC is only valid after enough anesthetic has been loaded into the body that the CNS is saturated and the CNS partial pressure of the agent is in equilibrium with the alveolar partial pressure

7. Pharmacokinetics
   (a) The time required to establish anesthesia is inversely proportional to water solubility—that is, **higher potency agents with lower water solubility induce anesthesia more rapidly**
   (b) Increasing the concentration of agent in inspired air proportionately increases the rate of transfer of agent into the bloodstream, thereby making induction of anesthesia faster

(c) Increasing the patient's ventilation also makes induction faster

(d) Conversely, **increasing the cardiac output SLOWS the induction of anesthesia**

(1) ↑ cardiac output → ↑ pulmonary arterial flow

(2) At a constant delivery of anesthetic agent, increasing blood flow allows more anesthetic to dissolve into the blood, causing a decrease in partial pressure or gas tension, thus reducing the driving force to establish an anesthetic partial pressure in the brain

(e) The greater the difference between venous and arterial concentrations of anesthetic, the longer it takes for equilibrium to be established, and the longer induction will take—this is particularly a problem with water-soluble agents

(f) Elimination of anesthetic works exactly opposite to induction of anesthesia—water-soluble agents take longer to eliminate

(g) The majority of elimination occurs via exhalation from the lungs, but some compounds do undergo metabolism

B. Ideal anesthetic agent

1. The ideal agent, which does not exist, would rapidly induce loss of consciousness, skeletal muscle relaxation, analgesia, and amnesia at concentrations that are not toxic

2. In addition, lack of flammability is a desirable trait

C. Inhalational anesthetic agents (see Table 5.2)

Table 5.2 Inhalational Anesthetics

Drug	Pharmacology
nitrous oxide (N_2O)	• Very low water solubility → rapid induction and recovery • MAC >100% (even 100% N_2O will not induce anesthesia in 50% of patients) • "Balanced anesthesia" = use of N_2O in combination with other agents, thereby allowing ↓ concentration of other agents that are toxic at higher doses • N_2O has no cardiovascular complications, excellent anesthetic, rapid acting, and not flammable—very commonly used

(Continued)

Table 5.2 (Continued)

Drug	Pharmacology
halothane	• Fairly rapid induction and recovery—slightly slower than N_2O • 15–20% metabolized by liver • Incomplete anesthetic, causes minimal anesthesia or neuromuscular blockade • Causes respiratory & myocardial depression and vasodilation → hypotension • Arrhythmogenic in presence of catecholamines, so not useful for pt on pressors • Can cause massive hepatic necrosis and malignant hyperthermia • Increases risk of malignant hyperthermia if used with succinylcholine • Not commonly used in adults, must be combined in "balanced anesthesia"
enflurane	• Similar to halothane, but produces some neuromuscular blockade • Less arrhythmogenic, so more appropriate than halothane for pt on pressors • Has minimal hepatotoxicity
isoflurane	• An isomer of enflurane, less soluble in blood → very rapid induction/emergence
desflurane	• Even less soluble in blood than isoflurane, minimal hepatic metabolism • Very safe drug as well, very commonly used clinically
sevoflurane	• Similar to desflurane but odor is less pungent, more acceptable to pts • Mild decrease in cardiac contractility, very commonly used clinically
ether & diethyl ether	• Not used anymore—flammable, explosive, water soluble, irritating to respiratory mucosa, myocardial depressant, vasodilator • However, both allow complete induction of anesthesia

1. Most inhalational agents fall short of the ideal agent
2. Balanced anesthesia
   (a) In combinations of more than one agent, the benefits of each agent can be exploited
   (b) Also, two agents toxic at high % administration can be combined at half-doses to allow additive effects of anesthesia without additive toxicity
D. Intravenous anesthetic agents (see Table 5.3)

Table 5.3 Intravenous Anesthetics

Drug	Pharmacology
Barbiturates	
thiopental	• GABA-mimetic, highly lipid soluble → extremely rapid anesthesia induction
	• Initial tissue distribution is proportional to distribution of blood flow, but redistribution occurs until the drug is in equilibrium in all tissues in the body
	• Slow metabolism, so continued administration can lead to drug buildup
	• Causes unconsciousness and amnesia, but not analgesia or skeletal muscle relaxation, so must be combined with other agents
	• Major toxicities include respiratory and myocardial depression, leading to decreased cardiac output and reflex tachycardia, dangerous in ischemia
Benzodiazepines	
diazepam	• Mechanism is binding to GABA receptor (all benzodiazepines work this way)
	• Causes unconsciousness & amnesia but no analgesia or skeletal muscle relaxation—must be used in combination with analgesics
	• Long elimination half-life, so emergence from anesthesia is slow
midazolam	• Much more rapid onset and emergence
Opioid Analgesics	
morphine	• Neuroleptanalgesia (useful for short procedures)
	⇒ Low dose opioids → pt not unconscious but is completely uninterested and detached from the environment, can respond to commands and communicate

(Continued)

Table 5.3 (Continued)

Drug	Pharmacology
	⇒ When combined with general anesthetics to induce complete unconsciousness, this is termed neuroleptanesthesia
	• Opioid anesthesia
	⇒ Higher dose opioids, causing loss of responsiveness
	⇒ Useful in major surgery for pts with depressed myocardial function
	⇒ Complete respiratory failure is a common side effect; intubate pts
fentanyl	• Much more potent and rapid acting than morphine
	• Fentanyl + droperidol is a common combination for neuroleptanalgesia
ketamine	• Highly lipophilic, metabolized by liver, excreted in urine & bile
	• Ketamine is a PCP derivative, and induces "dissociative anesthesia," a trancelike state in which pt appears to be awake but does not respond to stimuli
	• The drug causes profound analgesia and amnesia, can cause psychotic reactions
	• It is the ONLY IV anesthetic that causes cardiovascular stimulation, and does not cause respiratory depression
	• Also increases cerebral blood flow, and can cause ↑ intracranial pressure
propofol	• The most rapidly redistributed & eliminated IV agent, shortest duration of action
	• Causes unconsciousness and amnesia without analgesia or skeletal muscle relaxation, so must be combined in balanced anesthesia
	• Causes more respiratory and cardiovascular depression than barbiturates
etomidate	• Causes unconsciousness in seconds via GABA-like mechanism
	• Minimal cardiovascular or respiratory depression
	• Useful for rapid sequence induction prior to emergent intubation

6. ENDOCRINE DRUGS

I. Autacoids (see Table 6.1)

A. Autacoids are local-acting hormones

B. Prominent examples include eicosanoids, bradykinin, serotonin, histamine, nitric oxide

C. Eicosanoids (see Figure 6.1)

1. **All are derived from arachidonic acid**, which is formed via phospholipase A degradation of membrane phospholipids

2. Lipoxygenase converts arachidonic acid to the leukotrienes (LTs)

   (a) LTs induce potent vasoconstriction, increase vessel permeability, cause bronchoconstriction, and induce platelet aggregation

   (b) LTC, LTD, and LTE constitute the slow-reacting substance of anaphylaxis (SRS-A), the end-effector of anaphylactic, IgE reactions

   (c) LT antagonists (see Figure 6.1)

      (1) Zileuton inhibits 5-lipoxygenase, inhibiting leukotriene formation

      (2) Zafirlukast prevents the formation of LTD and E

      (3) Montelukast competitively inhibits the LTD receptor

3. Cyclooxygenase (COX) converts arachidonic acid to prostaglandin G (PGG)

   (a) COX-1 isoform is constitutively expressed in many cell types

   (b) COX-2 isoform is upregulated in immune cells during inflammation

4. Prostaglandins

   (a) Thromboxane synthetase converts PGH to thromboxane A (TXA)

   (b) **PGE and PGI cause vasodilation, but PGE and PGF cause smooth muscle constriction** in parenchymal organs

   (c) PGE also inhibits gastric acid secretion, increases glomerular filtration by vasodilating the proximal renal arterioles, and promotes GI motility

   (d) **PGE and PGI cause bronchodilation, but PGF and TXA cause bronchoconstriction**

   (e) PGE and PGI inhibit platelet aggregation

   (f) PGE and PGI maintain patency of ductus arteriosus after birth

Table 6.1 Autacoids

Drug	Characteristics
Eicosanoids	
LT antagonists	• Useful adjuncts for asthma, allowing steroid dose reduction
dinoprostone	• PGE analog, vaginal suppository → abortifacient
dinoprost	• PGF analog, intra-amniotic injection → abortifacient
carboprost	• Synthetic PG analog, IM injection → abortifacient
misoprostol (Cytotec)	• Oral PGE analog → ↓ gastric acid, ↑ mucus & HCO_3^-, ↑↑↑ diarrhea • Reduces ulcer incidence when used with NSAIDs
Kinin-Active Agents	
epoprostenol	• IV prostaglandin E causes vasodilation, indicated for severe pulmonary hypertension
treprostinil	• Requires central line with constant infusion via pump, risks of line infection and DVT • Similar to epoprostenol but administered SQ
aprotinin	• Kallikrein inhibitor; may decrease inflammation in pancreatitis and burns
ACE inhibitors	• Bradykinin is degraded by angiotensin converting enzyme (ACE) • ACE inhibitors prevent degradation of bradykinin, which contributes to the cough associated with ACE inhibitors and helps ↓ BP

Serotonin-Active Agents			
Drug	Receptor	Agonist/ Antagonist	Effect
buspirone	5-HT$_1$	Agonist	Anxiolytic
sumatriptan almotriptan eletriptan frovatriptan naratriptan rizatriptan	5-HT$_1$	Agonist	Antimigraine via vasoconstriction
methysergide cyproheptadine	5-HT$_2$	Antagonist	Antimigraine via vasoconstriction

Table 6.1 (Continued)

Drug	Receptor	Agonist/ Antagonist	Effect
Serotonin-Active Agents			
ondansetron granisetron palonosetron	5-HT$_3$	Antagonist	Antiemetic via chemoreceptor blockade
metoclopramide	5-HT$_4$	Agonist	Antiemetic via promotility & D$_2$ blockade
cisapride	5-HT$_4$	Agonist	Antiemetic via promotility, not used anymore due to drug interactions
tegaserod	5HT$_4$	Agonist (partial)	Activates receptors in the GI tract resulting in increased motility and relief of constipation and irritable bowel syndrome
Histamine-Active Agents			
catecholamines	<ul><li>β_2 agonism $\rightarrow \uparrow$ cAMP $\rightarrow \downarrow$ release of histamine from white blood cells and counteracts histamine's bronchoconstriction and $\uparrow$ vessel permeability</li></ul>		
methylxanthines	<ul><li>Inhibit cAMP phosphodiesterase $\rightarrow \uparrow$ cAMP $\rightarrow \downarrow$ histamine release</li></ul>		
cromolyn sodium	<ul><li>Stabilizes mast cell & basophil membranes $\rightarrow \downarrow$ histamine release</li><li>Useful in mild asthma—note: it's not a bronchodilator!</li></ul>		
H$_1$-blockers	<ul><li>1st generation</li><ul><li>$\Rightarrow$ diphenhydramine, chlorpheniramine, hydroxyzine, and astemizole are all useful as anti-itching and antiallergy medications</li><li>$\Rightarrow$ Due to antimuscarinic effects, they cause somnolence and may be used as hypnotics, and they all can cause some degree of urinary retention</li></ul><li>2nd generation</li></ul>		

(Continued)

ENDOCRINE DRUGS

Table 6.1 (Continued)

Drug	Characteristics
H$_2$-blockers	⇒ loratadine, fexofenadine, cetirizine, and azelastine (nasal spray) are less sedating and now used 1st line for seasonal allergies
	• Used as antacids (see Figure 7.1, Table 7.1)
Nitric Oxide Agents	
nitrates sildenafil tadalafil vardenafil	• All inhibit phosphodiesterase 5, resulting in prolonged nitric oxide mediated vessel relaxation and improved erectile function—should not be combined with nitrates or fatal cardiac events can occur
	• Because sildenafil crosses the threshold for also being a competitive inhibitor of PDE6, it can cause visual disturbances, most commonly blue-halo vision, tadalafil is very similar to sildenafil but does not inhibit PDE6 and has no visual side effects
	• Tadalafil has a much longer half-life (18 h vs. 4–5 h with others), so effect lasts for 1–2 days
Substance P-Active Agents	
capsaicin cream	• Depletes pain nerve endings of substance P
	• Used for topical treatment of arthritis pain or neuropathic pain
aprepitant	• a substance P receptor antagonist that acts as an antiemetic, augments actions of serotonin antagonists

D. Kinins
   1. Small polypeptides derived from plasma kininogen via action of kallikrein enzymes
   2. Potent vasodilators, increase microvascular permeability → ↓ BP → reflex ↑ HR
   3. Also cause smooth muscle constriction → bronchoconstriction, ↑ GI motility
   4. In inflammatory responses kinins → pain, edema, leukocyte accumulation
E. Serotonin (5-hydroxytryptamine = 5-HT)
   1. Causes GI motility, pain, itching, edema, and has protean effects on the cardiovascular system and in the CNS

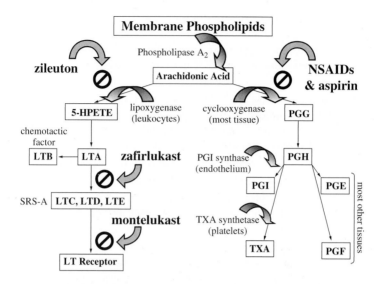

Figure 6.1 Eicosanoid Pathway
Eicosanoid synthesis begins with the breakdown of inner membrane phospholipids by phospholipase A_2 and the liberation of arachidonic acid. Arachidonic acid is then shunted in one of two directions. The enzyme 5-lipoxygenase converts arachidonic acid to 5-hydroperoxyeicosatetraenoic acid (5-HPETE), which then is converted into leukotriene A (LTA). When the action of lipoxygenase is inhibited by the antiasthma agent zileuton, formation of LTA is inhibited. LTA can be sequentially converted to LTC, LTD, and LTE, the three of which constitute the slow-reacting substance of anaphylaxis (SRS-A). SRS-A is one of the most potent mediators of bronchoconstriction and systemic vasodilation known. The antiasthma drug zafirlukast binds to specific receptors, which inhibits conversion of LTA to SRS-A. Another antiasthma medicine, montelukast, competitively inhibits the binding of LTD to its receptor. Conversely, arachidonic acid is converted to prostaglandin G (PGG) by the enzyme cyclooxygenase (COX). Aspirin irreversibly inhibits COX, whereas NSAIDs mediate reversible inhibition. PGG is converted to PGH, which can then be converted either to the vasodilators PGE or PGI (also called prostacyclin) or to the vasoconstrictors PGF and thromboxane A (TXA). PGI is exclusively formed in endothelium, and platelets make TXA.

2. Serotonin-active agents can be agonists or antagonists of serotonin receptors
3. Migraine headaches
    (a) **Serotonin 1 (5-HT$_1$) receptors cause vasoconstriction, whereas 5-HT$_2$ receptors cause vasodilation**
    (b) One mechanism to prevent or treat migraines is to decrease cerebral blood flow
    (c) This can be either by 5-HT$_1$ agonism or 5-HT$_2$ antagonism— 5-HT$_1$ agonism appears to be far more effective

    4. 5-HT_3 receptors stimulate vomiting in the CNS, so antagonists are used as antiemetics

    5. 5-HT_4 receptors stimulate gastrointestinal motility, so agonists are used to increase motility in gastroparesis or other conditions

F. Histamine

    1. Causes arteriolar vasodilation but pulmonary vein constriction, increases vascular permeability resulting in tissue edema, bronchoconstriction, ↑ GI motility, and reflex tachycardia, and has direct positive chronotropic and inotropic cardiac effects

    2. Also stimulates pain and itching and gastric acid secretion

    3. The key end-stage effector of all allergic reactions

    4. cAMP in the cytoplasm inhibits histamine release and causes bronchodilation, so stimulators of cAMP antagonize histaminergic effects

    5. Histamine uses two receptors, H_1 and H_2

        (a) **H_1 mediates the allergic effects of histamine**

            (1) H_1-blockers are useful for seasonal allergies (typically newer generation antihistamines that are less sedating), allergic rhinitis, drug allergies, anaphylactic reactions, and as premedication for blood transfusions

            (2) Older H_1-blockers tend to have anticholinergic effects, which cause side effects such as drowsiness, dry mouth, urinary retention

            (3) These older H_1-blockers are often used because of these side effects, for example, as sleeping pills and motion-sickness pills

        (b) **H_2 stimulates gastric acid production** (see Table 7.1, Figure 7.1 for H_2-blockers)

G. Nitric oxide

    1. Nitric oxide is a small, lipophilic molecule that easily diffuses across biological membranes

    2. Nitric oxide is unstable in oxygenated aqueous solution (half-life = 3–5 sec)

    3. Also called endothelium-derived relaxation factor (EDRF), nitric oxide is produced and liberated by endothelial cells and causes local smooth muscle relaxation → vasodilation

    4. **Bradykinin, histamine, arachidonic acid, acetylcholine, and other biological vasodilators all act by induction of formation of nitric oxide in endothelium**

    5. Nitric oxide is synthesized in endothelial cells by the enzyme nitric oxide synthase, which oxidizes L-arginine to nitric oxide + L-citrulline

6. Nitric oxide is also used by some neurons in the CNS as a neurotransmitter and is produced in massive quantities by leukocytes during inflammation, because nitric oxide can combine with oxidizers such as superoxide to form peroxynitrite (ONOO⁻), which is toxic to microbes

7. **Nitrate drugs, such as isosorbide dinitrate, nitroglycerin, and nitroprusside all contain nitric oxide in a bound form and work by steadily releasing nitric oxide in the bloodstream**

8. Nitric oxide diffuses across cell membranes and binds to intracellular guanylyl cyclase in smooth muscle cells, activating production of cyclic GMP (cGMP), which then decreases intracellular calcium levels and interferes with myosin light chain kinase → smooth muscle relaxation

9. Nitric oxide also prevents platelet aggregation

II. Pituitary/Hypothalamic Hormones (see Table 6.2)

Table 6.2 Pituitary Hormone Analogs & Antagonists

Drug	Characteristics
leuprolide	• Pulsatile dosing → ovulation in pts with central amenorrhea • Continuous dosing → suppress growth of endometriosis and prostate cancer
somatotropin	• ↑ muscle mass in pts with AIDS or cancer-associated wasting
octreotide	• A somatostatin analog with a long half-life • Used to prevent GI bleeding from varices in portal hypertension • Used to treat diarrhea in VIPoma and symptoms from carcinoid syndrome
bromocriptine	• Dopamine receptor agonist → inhibit prolactin secretion, shrink prolactinoma • Dosed daily and causes vomiting, hallucinations, postural hypotension
cabergoline	• Similar to bromocriptine, but dosed twice per week and much better tolerated

(*Continued*)

Table 6.2 (Continued)

Drug	Characteristics
phenothiazines	• Dopamine receptor antagonists used as antipsychotics or antiemetics, cause gynecomastia and galactorrhea as side effects
vasopressin	• Used as IV push in pulseless ventricular tachycardia/fibrillation (1st-line agent with epinephrine per the year 2000 ACLS guidelines) • Used as IV drip as a pressor agent for hypotensive pts
desmopressin (DDAVP)	• Given intranasally, subcutaneously, or IV • Used to treat central diabetes insipidus and as a procoagulant in von Willebrand's disease or other disease of platelet dysfunction (e.g., renal failure)
oxytocin	• One drug name is "Pitocin," widely used to induce labor
goserelin	• A gonadotropin-releasing hormone analogue used to treat breast and prostate cancer and endometriosis by reducing estrogen and testosterone
abarelix	• Antagonizes GnRH receptors, suppressing LH and FSH release and reducing the production of testosterone • Used in palliative chemotherapy for advanced stage prostate cancer

A. Gonadotropin-releasing hormone (GnRH) (see Figure 6.2)
   1. Made in hypothalamus, induces release of follicle stimulating hormone (FSH) and luteinizing hormone (LH) from the pituitary
   2. GnRH is normally produced in a pulsatile fashion, therefore the recombinant GnRH protein must be given in pulsed dosing to stimulate FSH and LH release
   3. **Constant infusion actually suppresses FSH and LH release**
   4. Used for induction of ovulation in women with hypothalamic amenorrhea, but has short half-life so cumbersome to dose
   5. Leuprolide acetate
      (a) A GnRH analog, which has a longer half-life because of reduced metabolism
      (b) Used to induce ovulation in amenorrhea (pulsatile dosing), or to suppress hormone sensitive proliferative growth (e.g., endometriosis, prostate cancer)

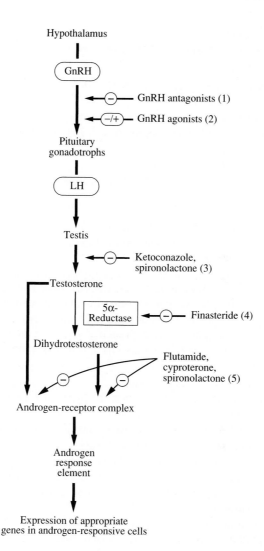

Figure 6.2 Control of androgen secretion and activity and some sites of action of antiandrogens

(1) Competitive inhibition of GnRH receptors; (2) stimulation (+, pulsatile administration) or inhibition via desensitization of GnRH receptors (–, continuous administration); (3) decreased synthesis of testosterone in the testis; (4) decreased synthesis of dihydrotestosterone by inhibition of 5α-reductase; (5) competition for binding to cytosol androgen receptors. (Redrawn from Katzung B. Basic & Clinical Pharmacology, 5th ed. Norwalk, Connecticut: Appleton & Lange, 1995:631.)

B. Somatotropin (growth hormone) has been used to correct dwarfism and to treat wasting in association with AIDS or malignancy

C. Somatostatin

1. A hypothalamic hormone, which inhibits somatotropin release from the pituitary

2. Also inhibits release of a variety of other hormones in the periphery, including glucagon, insulin, gastrin, and vasoactive intestinal peptide (VIP)

3. Octreotide

   (a) **A somatostatin analog that has a much longer half-life than somatostatin**

   (b) Variceal bleeding

      (1) **Principle use of octreotide is as a continuous drip to prevent gastrointestinal bleeding from esophageal varices**

      (2) The mechanism of this prevention has to do with reduction of portal pressures in portal hypertension, possibly via constriction of splanchnic vessels

   (c) Octreotide can also be used to prevent hormone-induced paraneoplastic disorders such as secretory diarrhea in VIPomas, and the symptoms of carcinoid syndrome

D. Prolactin

1. Prolactin secretion from the pituitary is regulated by the dopaminergic tract connecting the hypothalamus to the pituitary

2. **Dopamine secreted from the hypothalamus suppresses prolactin release from the pituitary**

   (a) Bromocriptine and cabergoline are dopamine receptor agonists used in the treatment of prolactinomas

   (b) These agents not only inhibit prolactin secretion but actually cause shrinkage of the tumor

3. Dopamine antagonists such as phenothiazines induce prolactin secretion → gynecomastia & galactorrhea

E. Vasopressin (antidiuretic hormone, ADH)

1. **Vasopressin binds to V_1 receptors on vascular smooth muscle → vasoconstriction**

2. **Vasopressin binds to V_2 receptors on the renal collecting ducts → ↑ H_2O resorption**

3. Vasopressin has a short half-life, but desmopressin (DDAVP) is a synthetic analog that is longer acting and has minimal V_1 activity (minimal pressor effects)

4. **Vasopressin can be used as a pressor in hypotensive pts and is listed in the year 2000 revised ACLS algorithm as a 1st-line agent (with epinephrine) for pts with pulseless ventricular tachycardia/fibrillation**

5. Desmopressin can be used to treat central diabetes insipidus (not nephrogenic, as the DDAVP requires functioning renal tubules for effect) and can also be used as a procoagulant in conditions of platelet dysfunction by inducing the release of von Willebrand's factor from endothelium (see section II: E)—it has minimal pressor effect

F. Oxytocin
   1. Secreted by posterior pituitary, stimulates milk secretion in lactating women
   2. Also induces uterine contractions during labor
   3. Given by IV drip to induce labor and to induce contractions postpartum to help decrease postpartum bleeding
   4. Can induce hypertension, and should not be used in pts on pressors

III. Adrenocorticosteroids (see Table 6.3)

A. Adrenal cortex is divided into three zones: zona glomerulosa, zona fasciculata, and zona reticularis

B. **Zona glomerulosa makes aldosterone (mineralocorticoid), fasciculata makes corticosteroids, reticularis makes testosterone (androgens)**

C. All steroids are lipophilic molecules synthesized from cholesterol

D. They work by diffusing across the cell membrane and binding to cytoplasmic receptors, and the complex of steroid/steroid receptor then diffuses into the nucleus where they stimulate transcription of a variety of genes

Table 6.3 Adrenocorticosteroid Analogs & Antagonists

Drug	Characteristics
spironolactone	• Directly antagonizes the aldosterone receptor, K^+-sparing diuretic
amiloride, triamterene	• Indirectly antagonize the aldosterone receptor, K^+-sparing diuretics
ACE inhibitors	• Block angiotensin II production, thereby blocking aldosterone production
fludrocortisone	• Replaces aldosterone in adrenal insufficiency

(Continued)

Table 6.3 (Continued)

Drug	Characteristics
aminoglutethimide	• Inhibits steroid synthesis in the adrenal gland • Used for medical adrenalectomy in Cushing's syndrome
metyrapone	• Inhibits glucocorticoid synthesis, but not other steroid synthesis • Used to assess integrity of adrenal axis, also used to suppress glucocorticoid production in Cushing's syndrome
ketoconazole	• Inhibits glucocorticoid synthesis, used in Cushing's syndrome
androgens	• Used to build muscle mass, treat hypogonadism, autoimmune diseases
cyproterone	• An antihirsutism drug, antagonizes androgens in the periphery
flutamide	• Antiandrogen used for prostate cancer
finasteride	• Topical use → ↑ hair growth, systemic use to shrink prostate in BPH

Glucocorticoids			
	Potency	Route	Indication
hydrocortisone	1	Oral, IV, topical, local injection	Dermatitis, adrenal insufficiency, local arthritis
prednisone	4	Oral	Asthma, systemic inflammation
prednisolone	5	Oral, IV, local injection	Asthma, systemic inflammation, local arthritis
methylprednisolone	5	Oral, IV	Asthma, systemic inflammation
dexamethasone	30	Oral, IV	CNS edema, systemic inflammation
triamcinolone	5	Topical, inhaled	Dermatitis, asthma (low potency inhaled)
betamethasone	30	Topical	Dermatitis
beclomethasone	Mid	Inhaled	Asthma, allergic rhinitis, sinusitis
budesonide	Mid	Inhaled	Asthma, allergic rhinitis, sinusitis
flunisolide	Mid	Inhaled	Asthma
fluticasone	High	Inhaled	Asthma

E. Zona glomerulosa agents

1. Aldosterone antagonists are used as potassium-sparing diuretics: spironolactone, amiloride, triamterene

2. ACE inhibitors block production of angiotensin II, thereby blocking production of aldosterone

3. Mineralocorticoid analogs are given, in conjunction with glucocorticoids, for adrenal insufficiency (Addison's disease), to supply the missing hormones: fludrocortisone is commonly used for this, but hydrocortisone has potent mineralocorticoid activity as well

F. Zona fasciculata

1. Glucocorticoids have a variety of effects on the body

   (a) ↑ blood glucose via ↑ gluconeogenesis & glycogenolysis

   (b) ↓ protein synthesis, ↓ bone formation, ↓ wound healing

   (c) ↑ lipolysis → ↑ serum lipids

   (d) ↓ inflammation & ↓ cell-mediated immunity by numerous mechanisms

      (1) Induce direct lympholysis at high doses

      (2) Suppress T-cell activation and proliferation

      (3) Suppress secretion of proinflammatory cytokines

      (4) ↓ chemotaxis of leukocytes, ↓ phagocytosis, ↓ intracellular killing of microbes

2. **The principal endogenous corticosteroid is cortisol, which by standard consensus is rated as having a relative anti-inflammatory potency of 1 and relative sodium retaining potency of 1**

3. **Hydrocortisone is a drug that is equivalent to cortisol** and is useful for physiologic replacement of adrenocorticosteroids in adrenal insufficiency and for topical use in any kind of dermatitis

4. A variety of synthetic glucocorticoids are available, all of which are more potent anti-inflammatory agents than hydrocortisone, but none of which are as potent at causing sodium retention

   (a) Prednisone

      (1) **The standard oral glucocorticoid in the United States**

      (2) Is fourfold more potent at anti-inflammation and fourfold less potent at causing sodium retention than hydrocortisone

      (3) Must be converted in the liver to prednisolone for effect

    (b) Prednisolone

       (1) Rarely used orally in the United States because of preference for prednisone

       (2) Can be given by local injection, which prednisone cannot (because prednisone must get to the liver for conversion to prednisolone for effect)

    (c) Methylprednisolone

       (1) **The preferred intravenous therapy for rapid, urgent anti-inflammatory effect**

       (2) Has five times the anti-inflammatory action of cortisol and essentially no sodium-retaining effect

    (d) Dexamethasone

       (1) **Because of its massive anti-inflammatory effect, it is the preferred agent to reduce CNS swelling due to tumors, inflammation, or trauma**

       (2) Has 30 times the anti-inflammatory action of cortisol and essentially no sodium-retaining effect

    (e) Topical agents

       (1) Hydrocortisone is the preferred low potency topical steroid (anti-inflammatory ratio of 1)

       (2) Triamcinolone is the preferred midpotency topical steroid (anti-inflammatory ratio of 5)

       (3) Betamethasone is the preferred high-potency topical steroid (anti-inflammatory ratio of 30)

    (f) Inhaled agents

       (1) Low potency = triamcinolone

       (2) Midpotency = beclomethasone, budesonide, flunisolide

       (3) High potency = fluticasone

5. Adverse effects from all glucocorticoids

    (a) **At steroid equivalents of ≥ 10 mg/day of prednisone for ≥ 4 weeks → significant ↑ risk of infections,** can have typical bacteria or a variety of atypical agents, including *Mycobacteria, Nocardia, Pneumocystis carinii, Aspergillus, Candida,* and others

    (b) Peptic ulcer formation and GI hemorrhage risk ↑ with steroids, especially if other risk factors are present (e.g., pt taking NSAIDs)

    (c) Can unmask glucose intolerance or cause frank diabetes and induce hypertension

    (d) Psychosis can develop rather acutely on steroid therapy, resolves with withdrawal

      (e) **Femoral head necrosis, cataracts, and severe osteoporosis develop with prolonged use**

      (f) **Cushing's syndrome** (buffalo hump, moon facies, abdominal striae, etc.) develops with prolonged use

      (g) **Adrenal insufficiency develops following sudden withdrawal**

6. Corticosteroid antagonists

    (a) Aminoglutethimide

      (1) Inhibits synthesis of steroids from cholesterol, causing medical adrenalectomy

      (2) Can be used in combination with ketoconazole to completely shut down steroid production in pts with Cushing's syndrome

    (b) Metyrapone

      (1) Inhibits 11-β-hydroxylase, which synthesizes cortisol, and therefore inhibits cortisol formation but not the formation of earlier precursors

      (2) Can be used as a test of adrenal function by looking for increases in the urinary levels of cortisol precursors, and can also be used to shut down cortisol production in Cushing's syndrome

      (3) Side effects include salt and water retention from shunting of steroids away from glucocorticoids and toward mineralocorticoids

    (c) Ketoconazole

      (1) An azole antifungal that inhibits glucocorticoid production at numerous steps in the synthetic pathway

      (2) Can be given with aminoglutethimide to suppress corticosteroid production in Cushing's syndrome

G. Zona reticularis

1. Makes androgens, principally dehydroepiandrosterone (DHEA), which is converted to testosterone peripherally

2. A variety of androgens, including testosterone, DHEA, and danazol, can be administered to improve muscle mass in patients with cancer, AIDS, or prolonged illness, to treat hypogonadism in males, and for some autoimmune diseases such as idiopathic thrombocytopenic purpura

3. Androgen inhibitors

    (a) Cyproterone inhibits androgen actions in the periphery and can be used as antihirsutism drug

    (b) Flutamide competitively antagonizes the testosterone receptor and has been used as an antiandrogen for prostate cancer

(c) Finasteride is an inhibitor of 5-α-reductase, the enzyme that converts testosterone to dihydrotestosterone (the more active form), and has been used topically as a hair-growth promoter for baldness and systemically as a therapy to shrink the prostate in benign prostatic hypertrophy

IV. Estrogens/Progestins (see Table 6.4)

A. Estrogens can be natural or synthetic

1. **Estrogens are given as hormone replacement therapy (HRT) for postmenopausal women, as 1st-line therapy for osteoporosis, as birth control pills in combination with progestins, or to treat infertility**

2. Estrogens suppress ovulation at high doses (lower doses required if progestins are included), stimulate endometrial proliferation, reduce LDL cholesterol, raise HDL cholesterol, may have other cardioprotective effects (controversial), predispose to thrombosis (hypercoagulable state), prevent bone resorption, and stimulate bone formation

Table 6.4 Estrogens & Progestins

Drug	Characteristics
estrogens	• Tx osteoporosis, oral contraceptives, hormone replacement • Adverse effects = deep vein thrombosis, endometrial cancer
clomiphene	• Induces ovulation, acts as an estrogen antagonist on the hypothalamus
tamoxifen	• An estrogen receptor agonist/antagonist • Mimics estrogen effects on bone, lipids, endometrium • Antagonizes estrogen effects on breast • Useful to prevent and treat breast cancer
raloxifene	• Similar to tamoxifen but lacks stimulatory effect on endometrium
progestins	• Contraceptives (alone or in combination with estrogens), appetite stimulants
Norplant	• A subcutaneous depot form of progestin that provides contraception for 5 yrs
RU-486	• A partial agonist/antagonist of progestin, provides postcoital contraception

3. Common side effects of estrogens include nausea, edema, weight gain, breast tenderness

4. **Estrogens do increase the risk of deep venous thrombosis, slightly increase the risk of endometrial cancer** (an effect completely neutralized by coadministration with progestins), and **high doses may slightly increase the risk of developing breast cancer** (this is controversial, and if they do increase the risk it is a very small increase)

5. Clomiphene citrate is an estrogen antagonist, which can stimulate ovulation by removing the feedback inhibition of estrogen on the hypothalamus (disinhibits the hypothalamus)

6. Partial agonist/antagonists (selective estrogen receptor modulators, SERMs)

   (a) Tamoxifen
      (1) Shares estrogen's agonist effects on endometrium, shares estrogen's cholesterol reducing capacity and bone density maintenance, but antagonizes estrogen receptors in the breast
      (2) It can be used as hormone replacement in patients with family history of breast cancer, and it **reduces the risk of breast cancer developing in patients at risk**
      (3) It is also used as adjunctive chemotherapy in patients who have had breast cancer to prevent recurrence or metastases

   (b) Raloxifene
      (1) A newer SERM, it is similar to tamoxifen but lacks tamoxifen's activity on the endometrium, suggesting it is safe in pts with a history of endometrial cancer
      (2) Like tamoxifen, raloxifene also reduces the risk of breast cancer, so raloxifene is also first line for this indication

B. Progestins

   1. **Progestins induce endometrial sloughing**, inhibit ovulation (especially in combination with estrogens), cause smooth muscle relaxation, and stimulate appetite

   2. They are used clinically as oral contraceptives either alone or in combination with estrogens, as hormone replacement therapy in combination with estrogens, and to stimulate appetite in cachectic individuals

   3. Medroxyprogesterone acetate is the preferred form to treat endometriosis or endometrial cancer and in combination with estrogens as hormone replacement therapy

4. A depo form of medroxyprogesterone is injected intramuscularly and provides contraception for approximately 12 weeks

5. Norplant is a time-released strip implanted subcutaneously, which slowly leaks the synthetic progestin, levonorgestrel, into the body, providing up to 5 years of continuous contraception

6. RU-486 is a progestin agonist/antagonist, which can be used for emergency postcoital contraception

V. Thyroid Hormones (see Table 6.5)

A. Thyroid hormone synthesis is regulated in part by an iodide pump in the thyroid

B. Thyroid stimulating hormone (TSH) stimulates the pump to uptake iodide, as do reduced levels of iodide

C. Inside the thyroid, thyroid peroxidase oxidizes iodide to iodine

D. Thyroid peroxidase then catalyzes the iodination of the organic precursor molecule, thyroglobulin, followed by the coupling of two iodinated thyroglobulin molecules to form one thyroid hormone molecule

E. Each thyroglobulin molecule has two potential sites for iodination

Table 6.5 Thyroid Agents

Drug	Characteristics
levothyroxine (T4)	• 1st-line therapy for hypothyroidism, monitor dose by TSH levels
T3	• Major indication is myxedema coma, not commonly used otherwise
methimazole	• Used for hyperthyroidism, inhibits organification of thyroxine • Takes 2–3 weeks for clinical effect
propylthiouracil	• Similar to methimazole, but also inhibits T4 to T3 conversion so can work more quickly • Should be given in thyroid storm for this reason
iodide	• Useful prior to surgery to shrink gland via feedback inhibition • Also given emergently for thyroid storm to prevent thyroid hormone release—never give iodine in thyroid storm until propylthiouracil is already on board
propranolol	• 1st-line agent for thyroid storm; can also be used in mild hyperthyroid

F. Coupling two thyroglobulin molecules with two iodines bound to each leads to formation of the T4 hormone (T4 refers to the presence of four iodines)

G. Coupling of one thyroglobulin that has two iodines and one thyroglobulin that has one iodine leads to the formation of T3 (T3 refers to the presence of three iodines)

H. T3 is far more potent but has a shorter half-life and shorter duration of action

I. **T4 is the dominant circulating form and is converted to T3 at peripheral sites by deiodination**

J. T4 can also be inactivated at peripheral sites by conversion to reverse T3 (rT3), a biologically null analog of T3

K. Hypothyroidism

   1. Synthetic T4 = levothyroxine is by far the most widely used thyroid hormone replacement agent in the world

   2. Synthetic T3 is also available, but is less widely used

   3. **Efficacy of dosing is monitored by checking TSH levels, which should normalize with thyroid replacement**

L. Hyperthyroidism

   1. There are three options to treat hyperthyroidism: surgical resection of the gland, radioiodine ablation, and medical thyroidectomy

   2. Surgery

      (a) Surgical resection is effective, but mandates lifelong thyroid hormone replacement

      (b) Free iodide may be administered before the surgery, as it feedback-inhibits thyroid gland growth, decreasing the vascularity of the gland and making it easier to resect

   3. Radioactive iodine

      (a) This is the most commonly used therapy

      (b) **It is highly effective, but if enough time elapses (≥ 20 to 30 yrs), everyone will become hypothyroid and require replacement**

   4. Medical thyroidectomy

      (a) Methimazole and propylthiouracil are the agents used

      (b) Both inhibit iodine organification in the thyroid, and thus take 3–4 weeks to have an antithyroid effect

      (c) Propylthiouracil also inhibits peripheral conversion of T4 to T3, and thus can have a small effect much earlier than methimazole

(d) Both require 1 to 2 yrs of medical therapy before thyroid function is normalized, and then after the drug is stopped up to 70% of pts relapse with hyperthyroidism

(e) Both cross the placenta, but propylthiouracil is more highly protein-bound in the serum and so crosses the placenta at lower levels—it is preferred in pregnancy

(f) Both agents can cause idiosyncratic agranulocytosis, rash, & lupus-like reactions

(g) **Despite all these negatives, these drugs are the only possible options to normalize a hyperactive thyroid,** leaving the patient without the need for lifelong thyroid hormone replacement therapy

M. Thyroid storm

1. Pts with thyroid storm cannot wait for radioactive iodine or medical thyroidectomy—they require immediate treatment in an intensive care unit

2. **First action is rapid administration of propranolol,** which not only will help control the severe autonomic hyperreactivity, thereby lowering heart rate, converting tachyarrhythmias to normal, and lowering blood pressure, but propranolol also inhibits the conversion of T4 to T3, thereby having a rapid, if weak, antithyroid effect

3. **Propylthiouracil should then be rapidly administered,** both because it inhibits T4 to T3 conversion and because it allows for a more rapid therapy to then be given—iodide

4. **Iodide-containing products (for example, sodium iodide, or iodinated organic products such as Telepaque) have a rapid feedback suppression on the thyroid gland (rapid = 2–3 days vs. 2–3 weeks for propylthiouracil), preventing thyroid hormone release, and they should be given after the propylthiouracil is on board—never give iodide before propylthiouracil is on board, because although iodide does feedback-inhibit the gland, the initial surge in iodine levels can acutely stimulate organification of thyroid hormone unless propylthiouracil is present to block this reaction**

VI. Hypoglycemic Agents

A. Insulin

1. Comes in many forms, each of which has its own duration of action and time to onset of action

2. In general the forms are broken into short-, intermediate-, and long-acting versions (see Table 6.6)
3. Insulin induces glucose uptake into muscle, liver, & brain, shuts down gluconeogenesis, shuts down glycolysis, induces potassium uptake into cells, inhibits lipolysis, & induces protein synthesis
4. Insulin secretion from the pancreas is stimulated by β-adrenergic receptors
5. Insulin is cleared by the kidney and has a markedly prolonged half-life in renal failure
6. Insulin is produced as a prohormone that is cleaved upon secretion, separating it from an inert fragment called the "C-peptide," which can be used as a marker of endogenous insulin secretion
7. Insulin is obviously used for diabetes, but is also used in acute hyperkalemia to cause a rapid intracellular shift of potassium—this is only a temporizing measure, as the potassium will soon leak back out of the cells
8. The major side effect is hypoglycemia
   (a) **Hypoglycemia induces neuroglycopenic and autonomic responses**
      (1) **Neuroglycopenic responses include presyncope or syncope, confusion**
      (2) **Autonomic responses include tremor, anxiety, palpitations, sweating**, and these can be blunted by β-blocker therapy or by very tight glucose control
   (b) Can be caused by too high a dose, worsening renal failure leading to buildup of levels of insulin in the body, infection, or liver failure (which cause hypoglycemia independent of insulin), or by concomitant oral hypoglycemic therapy

Table 6.6 Insulin Preparations

Type	Onset (hrs)	Peak (hrs)	Duration (hrs)
insulin lispro	1/4–1/2	1–2	4–8
regular insulin	1/2–1	1–2	6–8
semilente (zinc-conjugate)	1/2–1	1–2	12–16
NPH insulin	1–2	8–12	20–24
lente (zinc-conjugate)	1–2	8–12	20–24
protamine zinc insulin	3–4	8–12	36

9. Other side effects include stimulation of anti-insulin antibodies, which decrease the half-life of insulin, and lipodystrophy at the site of injection

B. Oral hypoglycemic agents (OHAs) (see Table 6.7)

1. Sulfonylureas

(a) Sulfa-derivative drugs, which cross-react in sulfa-allergic pts

(b) **Stimulate direct release of insulin from pancreatic cells and thus are not effective agents in pts with Type I diabetes** (who have no β cells left in their pancreas)

(c) First-generation agents, including chlorpropamide, acetohexamide, and tolbutamide, are rarely used now—chlorpropamide has an extremely long half-life, so hypoglycemia caused by chlorpropamide can last > 48 hours and requires prolonged hospitalization

Table 6.7 Oral Hypoglycemic Agents

Drug	Characteristics
sulfonylureas	• Stimulate insulin secretion from pancreas • Induce weight gain and can cause hypoglycemia
metformin	• Stimulates synthesis of insulin receptors, inhibits gluconeogenesis • Promotes weight loss, minimal risk of hypoglycemia, risk of lactic acidosis in pts with renal failure or congestive heart failure • Should be held in patients undergoing imaging studies with contrast (e.g., CT scan or cardiac catheter)
thiazolidinediones (e.g., pioglitazone & rosiglitazone)	• Increase tissue sensitivity to insulin • May cause liver toxicity, do cause peripheral volume expansion • Contraindicated in heart failure & can cause new onset heart failure
α-glucosidase inhibitors (e.g., acarbose miglitol)	• Inhibit absorption of carbohydrates • Hypoglycemic effect is weak, but low risk of hypoglycemia
meglitinides (e.g., repaglinide nateglinide)	• Drugs work like sulfonylureas but insulin is stimulated only in the presence of glucose, theoretically reducing risk of hypoglycemia

    (d) Second-generation agents include glyburide, glipizide, and glimepiride

    (e) All sulfonylureas tend to cause weight gain, and thus may not be ideal 1st-line agents for obese diabetics

2. Biguanides

    (a) Metformin is the only currently available drug in this class

    (b) Phenformin was taken off the market due to its propensity to induce fatal lactic acidosis—metformin can also induce lactic acidosis but it is much less common

    (c) **Metformin has two major mechanisms of action: it upregulates insulin receptors (makes the insulin more efficient), and it inhibits gluconeogenesis**

    (d) Because it does not induce insulin secretion, it is much less likely to cause hypoglycemia than sulfonylureas (unless it is combined with insulin or sulfonylureas!)

    (e) **Metformin actually induces mild weight loss, and so is an ideal 1st-line agent for obese diabetics**

    (f) Metformin is secreted by the kidneys, and renal failure is the major risk factor for metformin-induced lactic acidosis

    (g) Metformin is contraindicated in patients with renal failure or congestive heart failure

3. Thiazolidinediones

    (a) New class of agents that works by increasing tissue sensitivity to insulin

    (b) Troglitazone was the original drug in the class, but it has been pulled from the market due to multiple case reports of fulminant hepatic failure

    (c) Other agents include pioglitazone and rosiglitazone, which are new—thus far they do not appear to carry the risk of liver failure, although hepatic monitoring is warranted

    (d) The thiazolidinediones do cause peripheral volume expansion secondary to sodium retention via an unknown mechanism and can cause severe congestive heart failure—they are contraindicated in patients with heart failure or other disease (e.g., valve disease), which makes patients susceptible to heart failure

4. α-glucosidase inhibitors

    (a) Block action of α-glucosidase in the brush border of the intestinal microvilli

    (b) Interferes with carbohydrate uptake, blocking postprandial hyperglycemia

    (c) Major side effects are gassiness and bloating

5. Meglitinides
   (a) Represented by repaglinide and nateglinide
   (b Unlike sulfonylureas, they stimulate insulin only in the presence of glucose—although this theoretically reduces the risk of hypoglycemia, the effect is modest clinically

VII. Lipid Agents (see Table 6.8 and Figure 6.3)

A. Binding resins
   1. Cholestyramine and colestipol exchange chloride ions for bile salts in the GI tract, causing increased excretion of bile acids
   2. The loss of bile acids stimulates the enzyme 7-hydroxylase to degrade cholesterol in order to form more bile acids

Table 6.8 Lipid Agents

Drug	Characteristics
cholestyramine & colestipol	• Decreases plasma cholesterol levels, no effect on triglycerides • Binds to other drugs in the GI tract, ↓ absorption
niacin	• Most effective triglyceride-lowering agent, cholesterol reduction is modest • Cutaneous flushing occurs in everyone unless dose titrated up slowly
clofibrate	• Inhibits lipoprotein lipase → ↓ triglyceride levels
gemfibrozil	• Potent reducer of triglycerides, slight cholesterol-reducing effects • Combination with HMG-CoA reductase inhibitors → myositis
HMG-CoA reductase inhibitors	• Most effective cholesterol-lowering agents available • Fatal rhabdomyolysis may occur—cerivastatin withdrawn from market due to risk • Also ↑ HDL and ↓ triglycerides • Have been shown to reduce mortality from myocardial infarction & stroke • Watch for myositis or hepatitis developing on therapy
ezetimibe	• Inhibits absorption of cholesterol in the gut, additive effect with HMG-CoA reductase inhibitors

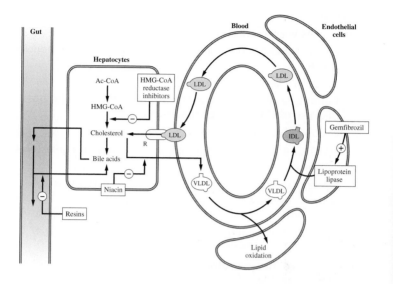

Figure 6.3 Mechanism of lipid-lowering agents
(Redrawn from Bhushan V, Le, T. First Aid for the USMLE Step 1:2005. New York: McGraw-Hill, 2005:319; originally adapted with permission from Katzung BG, Trevor AJ. USMLE Road Map: Pharmacology, 1st ed. New York: McGraw-Hill: 56.)

   3. The resins also bind to medications in the GI tract and can prevent their absorption

B. Niacin

   1. Inhibits triglyceride synthesis → ↓ VLDL → ↓ LDL

   2. Most effective at reducing triglyceride levels—**the most effective triglyceride reducing agent available**

   3. Cholesterol reduction does occur but is more modest, and HDL levels go up

   4. Commonly causes cutaneous flushing, which is lessened by slow titration of dose

C. Clofibrate

   1. Stimulates lipoprotein lipase → ↑ removal of VLDL from serum

   2. Lowers plasma triglycerides, also mildly decreases cholesterol levels

   3. Seldom used clinically, causes GI upset, gas, and may increase risk of hepatobiliary malignancy

D. Gemfibrozil
1. Inhibits VLDL production and enhanced VLDL clearance
2. Potent reducer of triglycerides, with slight cholesterol-reducing effects
3. Raises HDL levels
4. **Cannot be combined with HMG-CoA reductase inhibitors because of risk of inducing myositis**

E. HMG-CoA reductase inhibitors
1. **HMG-CoA reductase is the rate-limiting step in cholesterol synthesis**
2. Decreased production of cholesterol → ↑ LDL receptors on hepatic cell surfaces → ↑ uptake of circulating LDL → ↓ serum LDL levels
3. Myositis and hepatitis are relatively common, especially if combined with gemfibrozil
4. **These are the most effective cholesterol-reducing medicines available**
5. They also mildly increase HDL levels and decrease triglyceride levels
6. **Several of these drugs have been shown to reduce the risk of dying from cardiac disease and stroke**
7. They appear to have anti-inflammatory actions as well
8. Examples include lovastatin, simvastatin, pravastatin, atorvastatin, and fluvastatin

F. Ezetimibe
1. First drug in a new class, inhibits cholesterol absorption from gut
2. Drug is adjunctive with HMG-CoA reductase inhibitors, additive effect

VIII. Calcium Agents (see Table 6.9)

A. **For acute hypercalcemia, the first and by far the most important thing to do is vigorously hydrate the patient: normal saline preferred**

B. **Once euvolemia is restored, then give loop diuretic (furosemide)—do not give diuretic until euvolemia restored or you will worsen the hypercalcemia by worsening the hypovolemia**

Table 6.9 Calcium Agents

Drug	Characteristics
IV fluids	• 1st-line therapy for acute hypercalcemia—normal saline preferred
loop diuretic	• Furosemide used to diurese away calcium once euvolemia restored
bisphosphonate (alendronate, pamidronate, risedronate, zoledronic acid)	• The most effective calcium-lowering agents • Indicated for osteoporosis and malignant hypercalcemia
calcitonin	• Rapidly lowers calcium, but not by much • Tachyphylaxis develops with prolonged use • Has potent analgesic properties for bone pain
glucocorticoids	• Only useful to lower calcium in pts with granulomatous dz or lymphoma
gallium nitrate	• Previously used for acute hypercalcemia, but too toxic and doesn't work well
plicamycin	• Previously used for acute hypercalcemia, but too toxic and doesn't work well
estrogen	• 1st line for prevention and Tx of osteoporosis
calcium	• Supplements should be given to all postmenopausal women
thiazides	• 1st line for BP reduction in pt at risk for or suffering from osteoporosis
calcitriol	• Vitamin D analog → ↑ calcium absorption in hypoparathyroidism & renal failure
cinacalcet	• A calcimimetic agent that lowers calcium in patients with secondary hyperparathyroidism from renal failure, also indicated in those with parathyroid cancer • It increases the sensitivity of the calcium-sensing receptor to activation by extracellular calcium, resulting in decreased PTH and calcium levels

C. Bisphosphonates

1. Highly effective stabilizers of bony matrix, coat the hydroxyapatite with a nonbiodegradable bisphosphonate shell, protecting the bone from osteoclasts

2. Alendronate is oral, used for osteoporosis

3. Zoledronic acid is the most effective drug in preventing complications of malignant bone mets, and lasts for 3–4 weeks prior to redosing, in contrast to 1 week for pamidronate and daily dose for others

4. **For acute hypercalcemia, pamidronate, risedronate, or zoledronic acid should be infused IV, these are by far the most effective calcium lowering agents, however it takes 48 hrs for clinical effect to be seen**

D. Calcitonin

1. Can be given IV, subcutaneous, or nasal inhalation

2. Has a rapid acting, but weak, effect on lowering serum calcium

3. **More importantly it has analgesic properties**, so is useful for malignancy associated with bone pain

4. Tachyphylaxis invariably develops with long-term use

F. Glucocorticoids are particularly useful for lowering hypercalcemia associated with granulomatous diseases (e.g., fungal, TB) or lymphomas, but are minimally effective in other conditions

G. Gallium nitrate and plicamycin (mithramycin) were both previously used therapies for acute hypercalcemia, but are very rarely used now because of severe toxicities and low efficacy

H. **Estrogens are 1st-line therapy both to prevent osteoporosis and to treat established osteoporosis**

I. Calcium supplements (>1200 mg/day) should be given to postmenopausal women

J. Thiazide diuretics are appropriate blood pressure–reducing agents in patients with low calcium or those at risk for osteoporosis, because they increase resorption of calcium, leading to increased calcium levels in the blood

K. Calcitriol is the activated form of vitamin D, which is necessary for calcium absorption, and is thus used to treat hypocalcemia from hypoparathyroidism or end-stage renal failure

7. GI AGENTS

I. Acid Therapy (see Figure 7.1, Table 7.1)

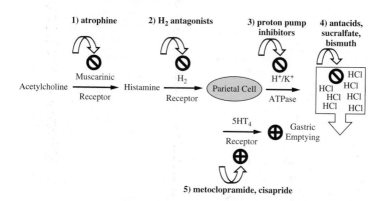

Figure 7.1 Antacid Therapy
Acid formation is amenable to pharmacologic intervention at five steps.
1) Atropine, or other anticholinergic therapy, is rarely used; however, surgical vagotomy of the stomach may be effective for patients with gastrinomas who develop ulcers refractory to standard therapy. **2)** H_2 antagonists are very commonly used and highly effective at suppressing acid production. **3)** Proton pump inhibitors (PPIs) offer by far the most powerful antacid therapy available. They can increase the pH in the stomach from 1 to 7 (neutral) and are 1st line for ulcer therapy and all severe conditions related to acid imbalance (e.g., bleeding gastritis, esophagitis). **4)** Direct antacids are useful for symptomatic relief, but they should NEVER be used in lieu of H_2-blockers or PPIs for patients with serious medical consequences of gastric acid imbalance. 5) Metoclopramide is most useful in patients with gastric hypomotility (e.g., diabetic gastroparesis). Cisapride is no longer available owing to toxic cytochrome p450 interactions with other drugs, which lead to widened QT and torsade de pointes.

Table 7.1 Acid Therapy

Drug	Activity	Clinical Indication/Characteristics
atropine	Antagonize muscarinic receptor	• Atropine not used clinically • Refractory ulcers (e.g., from gastrinomas) can be treated surgically by denervation of cholinergic fibers to the stomach
cimetidine, ranitidine, famotidine, nizatidine	Antagonize H_2 receptor	• Widely used as 1st-line Tx • Appropriate Tx for uncomplicated acid reflux or stress ulcer prophylaxis in the ICU • Cimetidine has more cytochrome p450 inhibition than others • All may be associated with drug-induced thrombocytopenia (controversial)
omeprazole, lansoprazole, pantoprazole, esomeprazole, rabeprazole	Antagonize H^+/K^+ ATPase pump	• By far most potent & effective acid blockers • Should be used for any patient with severe gastritis or reflux unresponsive to H_2-blockers, or for patients with ulcers or pathologic sequelae of GI acid (e.g., Barrett's esophagus)
antacids	Neutralize acid	• Useful for symptomatic relief, not sufficient for ulcer or gastritis Tx, or as preventive medicines for chronic reflux • Extremely safe, so available over the counter
metoclopramide, cisapride	5-HT_4 receptor agonism	• Metoclopramide rarely used as antacid, only useful in patients with decreased gastric motility (e.g., diabetic gastroparesis) • Cisapride no longer available because of severe p450 inhibition leading to cardiac arrhythmia if used with other drugs (e.g., erythromycin)

Table 7.1 (Continued)

Drug	Activity	Clinical Indication/Characteristics
sucralfate	Mucosal protectant	• Sucralfate polymerizes to form a gelatinous matrix at low pH, sticks to and protects exposed ulcers in the mucosa from acid • Only used as stress ulcer prophylaxis in the ICU, and should never be given jointly with an H_2-blocker or proton pump inhibitor because sucralfate requires acidity to polymerize
bismuth subsalicylate (Pepto-Bismol)	Mucosal protectant	• Coats exposed ulcers, protects from acid • Also direct toxicity to *H. pylori* • Like antacids, useful for symptomatic relief and is safe, so is available over the counter

II. Emesis Therapy (see Figure 7.2, Table 7.2)

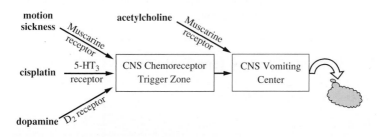

Figure 7.2 Antiemetic Therapy
Vomiting is principally regulated in the CNS chemoreceptor trigger zone. Muscarinic, serotonergic, and dopaminergic signals can trigger this response. Scopolamine is an anticholinergic drug with CNS effects, particularly useful for motion sickness. Ondansetron and granisetron are serotonergic antagonists ($5-HT_3$ antagonists) and are among the most powerful antiemetics available, especially for chemotherapy-induced nausea and vomiting. Dopamine antagonists, especially metoclopramide and prochlorperazine, are perhaps the most commonly used drugs to treat non–chemotherapy-associated nausea and vomiting.

GI AGENTS

Table 7.2 Therapy for Emesis

Drug	Receptor Activity	Clinical Indication
phenothiazines (prochlorperazine, promethazine)	Antagonize D_2	• Useful for any nausea/vomiting • 1st-line choice for most hospitalized patients
metoclopramide	Agonize $5\text{-}HT_4$, Antagonize D_2	• Particularly for nausea with dysmotility (e.g., diabetic gastroparesis)
ondansetron, granisetron, palonosetron	Antagonize $5\text{-}HT_3$	• Chemotherapy—the most effective drugs for this indication
atropine	Antagonize muscarinic	• Cholinergic toxicity
scopolamine	Antagonize muscarinic	• Motion sickness
diphenhydramine	Antagonize muscarinic	• Motion sickness
aprepitant	Substance P antagonist, enhances serotonin active agents	• Chemotherapy

III. Diarrhea Therapy (see Table 7.3)

Table 7.3 Therapy for Diarrhea

Drug	Mechanism
attapulgite (Kaopectate)	Physical coating of mucosa, absorbs water out of stool
diphenoxylate (Lomotil) *affects motility*	Activates opiate receptors in gut with minimal CNS effects
loperamide (Imodium)	Activates opiate receptors in gut, poorly absorbed so minimal side effects
bismuth subsalicylate (Pepto-Bismol)	Decreases fluid secretion into bowel, also direct antimicrobial properties, especially useful for infectious diarrhea

Note: Inflammatory diarrhea (e.g., bloody) should not be treated with antimotility agents, as this can increase contact of toxins with bowel wall, leading to worsening inflammation and possibly bowel perforation.

IV. Constipation Therapy (see Table 7.4)

Table 7.4 Therapy for Constipation

Drugs	Mechanism
Osmotic Laxatives	
magnesium sulfate, magnesium hydroxide, magnesium chloride, sodium phosphate, lactulose	Hypertonic solutions draw fluid into the bowel—lactulose is a synthetic disaccharide that cannot be absorbed
Bulk Laxatives	
bran, methyl cellulose	Nondigested, absorb water in the bowel lumen
Mucosal Stimulants	
cascara, castor oil, senna, bisacodyl	Stimulate bowel peristalsis
Fecal Softener	
docusate	A detergent, allows water to penetrate the stool

8. CARDIOVASCULAR DRUGS

I. Vasodilators (see Table 8.1)

A. Nitrates (see Figure 8.1)

1. **Molecules containing chemically coupled nitric oxide**
2. Work by steadily releasing nitric oxide into the vasculature
3. **Nitrates cause dilation of both arteries and veins → ↓ preload and afterload → ↓ myocardial O_2 demand, but effect on veins and preload is far greater than on arteries and afterload**

B. Calcium channel blockers

1. Prevent influx of calcium via L-type calcium channels found on muscle tissue
2. Vascular smooth muscle and cardiac muscle is more sensitive to calcium channel blockade than is smooth muscle found in other organs (e.g., airway, GI tract, uterus)
3. **Arterial smooth muscle is more sensitive than venous smooth muscle, and because of this, calcium channel blockers reduce afterload without markedly reducing preload, and thus without causing marked orthostatic hypotension**
4. **Two general classes of calcium channel blockers**
    (a) Dihydropyridines
    (1) All end in "-ine": e.g., nifedipine, amlodipine
    (2) **Much more selective effect on vasculature than on cardiac muscle**
    (3) Thus cause minimal decrease in cardiac contractility, and have only slight effects on automaticity of the SA and AV nodes and on conduction between them
    (4) **The results are marked arteriodilation → ↓ afterload → ↓ BP → autonomic reflex tachycardia**
    (5) **Because of the reflex tachycardia, dihydropyridines should be avoided in acute ischemia unless β-blockers are concurrently administered to blunt the reflex tachycardia**

Table 8.1 Vasodilators

Drug	Characteristics
Nitrates	
nitroglycerin	• Contains 3 nitrate groups (NO_2) bound to glycerin (also called glycerin trinitrate, see Figure 8.1) • Undergoes first-pass metabolism in the liver so cannot be given orally & its duration of action is very short (a few minutes) • Administered via IV drip, topical paste to skin, or via sublingual tablets • Primary indication is for acute ischemic chest pain (i.e., angina)
isosorbide dinitrate	• More stable than nitroglycerin, so longer lasting and can be given orally • Used for long-term therapy for chronic angina
nitroprusside	• A potent vasodilator used as an IV drip in hypertensive crises—not for angina (nitroglycerin preferred for angina) • Prolonged use can lead to cyanide toxicity (see Figure 8.1C)
Calcium Blockers	
dihydropyridines	• 2nd line for essential hypertension and heart failure • 1st line for acute coronary vasospasm (Prinzmetal's angina) • Avoid in acute ischemia due to reflex tachycardia (unless β-blockers are on board)—short-acting drugs shown to ↑ mortality in pts with coronary dz • Nimodipine is cerebral selective—1st line for subarachnoid hemorrhage to prevent coronary vasospasm
diltiazem	• 1st line for acute rate control of atrial fibrillation/flutter • Use cautiously in those with decreased ejection fraction • 2nd line to slow heart rate in ischemia if β-blockers are contraindicated • Do not combine with β-blockers because of risk of 3° block

Handwritten annotations next to dihydropyridines: Amlodipine / Felo / Nimo / Nife

(Continued)

Table 8.1 (Continued)

Drug	Characteristics
verapamil	• 1st line for acute rate control of atrial fibrillation/flutter • Contraindicated in those with decreased ejection fraction • Do not combine with β-blockers due to risk of 3° block
hydrazaline	• Direct arterio-dilator, 2nd line for heart failure (behind ACE inhibitor) • Must be combined with a β-blocker and diuretic
minoxidil	• Only used for severe, refractory hypertension • Must be combined with a β-blocker and diuretic • Beware of hair overgrowth!
ACE inhibitors	• 1st line for all patients with low ejection fractions (proven to ↓ mortality) • 1st line for all patients with postmyocardial infarction (proven to ↓ mortality) • 1st line for all diabetic patients and those with risks for vascular dz (proven to ↓ risk of stroke, myocardial infarction, death) • 1st line for all patients with proteinuria (↓ proteinuria) • Avoid in patients with ↑ baseline creatinine (> 2 mg/dL) and ↑ potassium
ATRAs	• Useful in patients intolerant of ACE inhibitors because of cough
Biotherapeutics	
nesiritide	• Recombinant human β natriuretic peptide, causes cGMP-mediated coronary and renal vasodilation, improving hemodynamics in heart failure—must be given in monitored setting due to risk of hypotension

   (b) Nondihydropyridines
      (1) There are two widely used nondihydropyridines: diltiazem and verapamil
      (2) **Diltiazem has an equivalent effect on vasculature and cardiac muscle, whereas verapamil has a greater effect on cardiac muscle than on vasculature**
      (3) **Thus diltiazem and verapamil are both useful to slow the heart rate** (via depression of SA and AV nodal

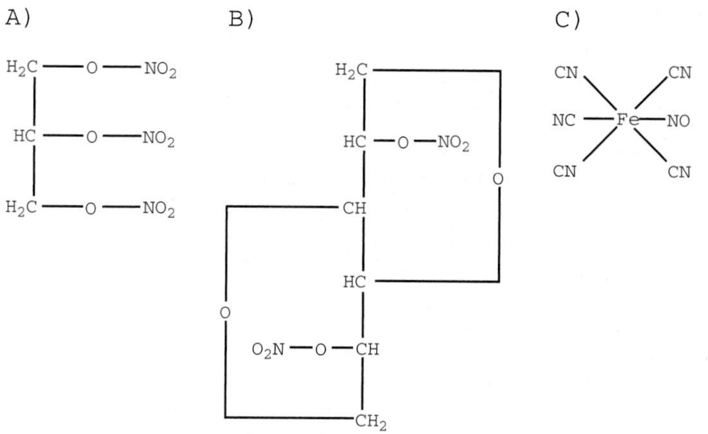

A)

B)

C)

Figure 8.1 Structure of nitrates
A. Nitroglycerin contains three molecules of nitrate (NO_2) esterified to a glycerin backbone. **B.** Isosorbide dinitrate contains two molecules of nitrate but is a more complicated, more stable ester. It can be administered orally and is longer lasting than nitroglycerin. **C.** Nitroprusside is an unstable inorganic nitrate that contains five molecules of cyanide (CN) and 1 molecule of nitric oxide that is not esterified. The half-life of nitroprusside is very short, and it must be administered as an IV drip. Prolonged use can lead to cyanide toxicity.

automaticity and conduction between them), but both can depress contractility → ↓ cardiac output

(4) These drugs should be avoided in heart failure due to the ↓ contractility

(5) **These drugs should not be combined with β-blockers or complete heart block can ensue**

C. Hydralazine

1. Mechanism of action unclear, **causes direct arteriolar vasodilation**

2. Like calcium blockers, causes minimal venodilation, and thus decreases afterload without affecting preload, so causes minimal orthostatic hypotension

3. **Has no negative chronotropic effects on heart, so causes marked reflex tachycardia and typically must be combined with a β-blocker to prevent this**

4. Short half-life, must be dosed three or four times per day, makes compliance difficult

D. Minoxidil

1. Opens potassium channel on smooth muscle → closure of calcium channels
2. **Only used for very severe, very refractory hypertension**
3. **Causes marked reflex tachycardia and fluid retention, so must be combined with both a β-blocker and a diuretic**
4. Topical version used as a hair-growth stimulator
5. Major side effect is diffuse hypertrichosis, making it especially awkward to use in women

E. Angiotensin converting enzyme inhibitors (ACE inhibitors)

1. Angiotensin converting enzyme converts angiotensin I to angiotensin II, which acts as a potent vasoconstrictor, stimulates catecholamine release, and induces sodium and fluid retention in the kidneys
2. **ACE inhibitors block conversion of angiotensin I to angiotensin II, but ALSO block the degradation of bradykinin,** which acts as a direct vasodilator
3. **The resulting increase in serum bradykinin can cause a distressing cough in some patients**
4. **Inhibition of bradykinin degradation can also lead to severe angioedema**
5. Angiotensin II also normally causes constriction of the efferent renal arterioles, so ACE inhibitors can also decrease glomerular perfusion pressure by causing dilation of efferent arterioles—this can lead to an alarming increase in creatinine in some patients
6. Angiotensin II also stimulates aldosterone synthesis, so ACE inhibitors can lead to hyperkalemia
7. Common ACE inhibitors include captopril, enalapril, benazepril, lisinopril, fosinopril, ramipril, quinapril, perindopril
8. One major difference between ACE inhibitors is the half-life
   (a) Because captopril has a short half-life, it is dosed three times per day, and thus acutely ill patients (e.g., hypertensive urgency or congestive heart failure) can rapidly be titrated up to the maximum tolerated dose
   (b) **Hence, captopril is the preferred agent for initiation of therapy in acutely ill individuals who need rapid reduction of afterload**
   (c) However, the other ACE inhibitors are dosed once or twice daily, so they are preferred for outpatient therapy

F. Angiotensin II receptor antagonists (ATRAs)

1. These agents work by blocking the binding of angiotensin II to its receptor

2. **They share many of the same properties as ACE inhibitors, but because they do not prevent the degradation of bradykinin, they do not cause a cough**—it is unclear if their blood pressure–reducing effects are affected by their lack of effect on bradykinin

3. Common ATRAs include losartan, candesartan, irbesartan, valsartan, eprosartan, olmesartan, telmisartan

G. Biotherapeutics

1. Novel drug, nesiritide, is recombinant human β natriuretic peptide

2. Mechanism is activation of guanylate cyclase in vascular smooth muscle cells → ↑ cGMP → smooth muscle relaxation and vasodilatation (both arterial and venous) → ↓ preload & afterload and ↓ myocardial oxygen demand

3. Nesiritide also improves glomerular filtration rate via afferent arteriole vasodilatation and efferent arteriole vasoconstriction

4. Drug must be given in monitored setting due to risk of hypotension

5. Indicated for decompensated CHF and shown to improve hemodynamics in the short term, **however, the drug may actually increase risk of death according to one meta-analysis** (JAMA 2005 293:1900-5)

II. Diuretics (see Figure 8.2)

A. Thiazide diuretics (see Table 8.2)

1. Inhibit sodium chloride resorption in the distal convoluted tubules, and water passively follows the salt into the tubules and is excreted

2. **Because they work distally, they have a lower intrinsic diuretic effect than drugs that work more proximally** (the magnitude of water loss is lower the more distal the diuretic works)

3. **Thiazides enhance calcium absorption, so are useful as diuretics in women at risk for osteoporosis, but should be avoided in patients with hypercalcemia**

4. **Thiazides can inhibit uric acid secretion in the proximal tubule, elevating serum uric acid levels, so use them carefully or not at all in pts with gout**

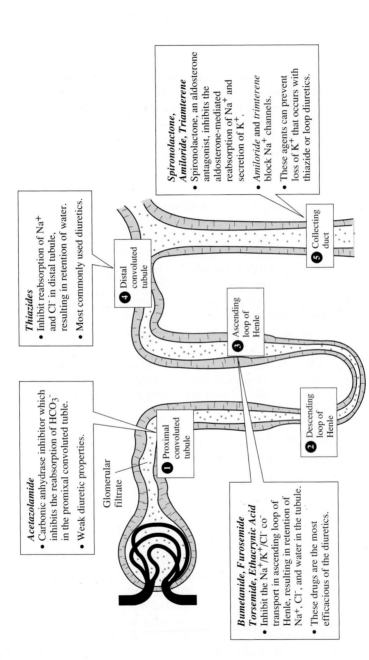

Figure 8.2 Major locations of ion and water exchange in the nephron, showing sites of action of the diuretic drugs (Redrawn from Howland RD, Mycek MJ, Harvey RA, Champe PC. Lippincott's Illustrated Reviews: Pharmacology, 2nd ed. Baltimore: Lippincott Williams & Wilkins, 2001:224.)

Table 8.2 Diuretics

Class (Drug)	Site of Action	Characteristics
thiazides (hydrochlorothiazide) *Half Life ~2.5hrs* *Chlorthalidone 47hrs!* *don't impact pts @ normal BPs, so should be fine*	Distal tubule	• Better blood pressure reducers than diuretics • Main use in essential hypertension (1st-line agent) • Increase calcium absorption so useful in women at risk for osteoporosis
loop diuretics *L→Anti-edema! can potentiate gout 2° to concentration of fluid loss* *Furosimide 60% BioAv 1.5hr Halflife* *Torsemide "to be pharmacists friend" 80% 3.5 hr* *Ethacrynic for SULFA-allergic*	Loop of Henle	• Most effective diuretics available • Poor antihypertensive effects • Major indications are heart failure, cirrhosis with ascites, renal failure with fluid overload, and ↑ Ca²⁺, *Anion overdose: I⁻, F⁻, Br⁻* • Furosemide is by far the most commonly used agent • All except ethacrynic acid contain sulfa moieties and cannot be given to sulfa-allergic patients
potassium-sparing diuretics (spironolactone, amiloride, triamterene, eplerenone) *Spironolactone & Eplerenone ↓ mortality in CHF pts! → by preventing remodeling in heart* *drug of choice for liver cirrhosis*	Distal tubule, collecting tubule	• Always used in combination with other diuretics—combination with thiazide for blood pressure and combination with furosemide for ascites • Spironolactone and eplerenone proven to decrease mortality in congestive heart failure • Prominent side effect of spironolactone is gynecomastia
carbonic anhydrase inhibitor (acetazolamide)	Proximal tubule	• Rarely used for diuresis because of metabolic toxicity • Indicated for glaucoma and high altitude illness
osmotic diuretic (mannitol)	Proximal tubule, loop of Henle	• Only indication is acute cerebral edema • Often seen in pathologic states (high serum glucose)

5. The antihypertensive effect of diuretics is not well correlated to their diuretic effect, and thiazides are potent reducers of blood pressure

6. **The major use for thiazides is in treatment of essential hypertension, in which they are considered 1st-line agents along with β-blockers**

7. Hyperuricemia, hyperglycemia (in diabetics), hypokalemia, and allergic reactions are the most common side effects—note that **thiazides have sulfa moieties and thus pts allergic to sulfa drugs should not be given thiazides**

B. Loop diuretics

1. Selectively inhibit sodium chloride resorption in the thick ascending limb of the loop of Henle by blocking the Na/K/Cl transporter on the luminal face of the loop

2. **Because they work more proximally than thiazides, they are much more effective diuretics—they have higher intrinsic activity**

3. **However, they are not very effective at reducing blood pressure unless the pt is volume-overloaded**

4. **Because the pump they inhibit is on the luminal face of the tubules, loop diuretics lose efficacy in patients with very low glomerular filtration rate—the drug must get into the tubules to block the transporter**

5. **Like thiazides, they can inhibit excretion of uric acid**, worsening hyperuricemia, but unlike thiazides they cause loss of calcium in the urine

6. Hypokalemia is a much bigger problem with loop diuretics than thiazides

7. Like thiazides, most **loop diuretics have sulfa moieties and should not be given to sulfa-allergic patients—ethacrynic acid is a non–sulfa-based drug that can be given to patients who are sulfa-allergic**

8. **Loop diuretics are primarily indicated for the diuresis of water in patients who are significantly volume-overloaded— these are the most effective diuretics available**

9. Principal side effects relate to excessive volume loss, hypokalemia, hypomagnesemia in nonmonitored patients, and sulfa reactions

C. Potassium-sparing diuretics

1. Act in the cortical collecting tubule and late distal tubule (distal to thiazides), and thus **have low intrinsic diuretic activity—that is, they are weak diuretics**

2. **These drugs directly or indirectly antagonize the effects of aldosterone**

3. **Spironolactone and eplerenone act as aldosterone receptor antagonists**, blocking sodium-potassium exchange in the distal tubule

4. **Amiloride and triamterene inhibit sodium transport in the collecting tubule, and because potassium secretion is linked to sodium uptake, they block the effect of aldosterone on sodium resorption and potassium excretion**

5. These diuretics can cause dangerous hyperkalemia if not monitored closely—they may be combined with thiazides for balanced electrolyte diuresis (e.g., hydrochlorothiazide/triamterene)

6. Their main use is in combination with other diuretics to prevent potassium loss

7. Spironolactone and eplerenone can be used as aldosterone antagonists in hyper-aldosterone states (e.g., Conn's syndrome) and have been **proven to reduce mortality in patients with severe congestive heart failure (CHF, mechanism unclear)**

8. Spironolactone can cause gynecomastia

D. Carbonic anhydrase inhibitors

1. Work primarily in the proximal tubule—**they are thus the most proximal-acting agents and have the highest intrinsic activity; however, they are not highly effective agents because the sodium and water trapped in the tubule get reabsorbed in the loop of Henle or distal tubules unless combined with other types of diuretics**

2. **Combinations of carbonic anhydrase inhibitors with loop or thiazide diuretics are extremely potent at inducing diuresis, but are also associated with metabolic derangements**

3. Carbonic anhydrase converts H_2CO_3 to $H_2O + HCO_2^-$, which is necessary for the proximal resorption of bicarbonate

4. Inhibition of carbonic anhydrase causes massive bicarbonate diuresis, leading to a hyperchloremic metabolic acidosis and massive potassium wasting

5. Because of the toxic potential, these drugs are only very rarely used as diuretics (ironically, they are TOO effective so they are not used)—however, they are occasionally used in a patient with a metabolic alkalosis

6. They can be used topically as eyedrops to treat glaucoma (inhibits aqueous humor formation in the eye), and they are indicated to prevent and treat acute high-altitude sickness caused by acute respiratory alkalosis

E. Osmotic diuretics

1. Because the proximal tubule and descending limb of the loop of Henle are freely permeable to water, osmotic agents that are not transported (that is, they stay in the tubules) draw water into the tubules, thereby promoting diuresis

2. **The major use of osmotic diuretics is in states of elevated intracranial pressure**, to attempt to draw water from the edematous brain by osmosis

3. Osmotic diuretics are often clinically seen in disease states—for example, in out-of-control diabetes and ketoacidosis, very high glucose levels in the serum cause glucose to spill into the urine faster than it can be reabsorbed in the tubules, leading to osmotic diuresis, dehydration, and eventual vascular collapse

III. Inotropes (see Table 8.3)

Table 8.3 Inotropes

Drug	Characteristics
digoxin	• Increases myocardial contractility with minimal increase in O_2 consumption • 1st line for heart failure (does NOT ↓ mortality, but does ↓ failure symptoms) • 1st line for long-term rate control in atrial fibrillation
milrinone amrinone	• Markedly increases myocardial O_2 demand with increased contractility • Used only for refractory cardiogenic shock
dopamine	• 1st-line inotrope for conditions of low SVR • Combined with dobutamine for cardiogenic shock
dobutamine	• 1st line for severe heart failure not associated with refractory hypotension • Must be combined with dopamine if refractory hypotension present
epinephrine	• Used as single-dose IV push in code blue • May be used as a drip in refractory cardiogenic shock • Markedly increases myocardial O_2 demand via ↑ HR, ↑ contractility
norepinephrine	• Often used as a pressor by ↑ SVR

A. Definitions

1. **An inotrope is an agent that increases myocardial contractility**

2. **A pressor is an agent that increases BP**

3. Some pressors are inotropes, but many pressors increase BP by increasing systemic vascular resistance (SVR), not by increasing myocardial contractility

B. Digoxin (see Table 8.3)

1. A relatively polar compound with a long half-life ($\approx$ 40 hrs) allowing once-a-day dosing

2. **Digoxin poisons the Na^+/K^+ ATPase antiporter pump in the sarcolemma, thereby preventing the uptake of potassium and export of sodium from the cell**

3. **Digoxin competitively binds to the potassium binding site on the ATPase, so digoxin binding is increased in hypokalemia and decreased in hyperkalemia**

4. Normally the Na^+/K^+ ATPase pumps sodium out of the cell, and the sodium then reenters the cell via a Na^+/Ca^{2+} antiporter, which pumps sodium back into the cell in exchange for calcium export from the cell

5. **Thus, by poisoning the Na^+/K^+ ATPase, digoxin causes a buildup of sodium in the cell and a deficiency of sodium outside of the cell, which prevents the export of calcium from the cell**

6. The result is an increase in intracellular calcium, which increases the actin-myosin cross-bridges $\rightarrow \uparrow$ myocardial contractility $\rightarrow \uparrow$ cardiac output

7. Digoxin often causes bradycardia by autonomic reflex ($\uparrow$ cardiac output $\rightarrow \downarrow$ HR to maintain BP) and by direct cholinomimetic effects on the SA and AV nodes

8. **Thus, digoxin causes minimal increase in myocardial oxygen consumption despite markedly improving cardiac performance**

9. **Digoxin does not decrease mortality in heart failure, but it does improve exercise tolerance and quality of life and decreases the frequency of hospitalization**

10. Because of its cholinomimetic effects on the AV node, it can also slow the ventricular response to atrial fibrillation

11. Adverse effects

    (a) **There is a small therapeutic window for digoxin**, and adverse effects are commonly seen at therapeutic doses

    (b) The principal adverse effect of digoxin is arrhythmia
- (1) Digoxin causes increased cardiac automaticity $\rightarrow$ premature ventricular contractions
- (2) Digoxin also slows cardiac conduction and slows conduction in the AV node
- (3) With decreased cardiac conduction and increased automaticity, reentrant supraventricular, junctional, and ventricular tachycardias occur

    (c) At high serum levels CNS & GI toxicity is prominent $\rightarrow$ hazy vision, yellow-tainted vision, headache, vomiting

    (d) **Note that because binding of digoxin to the ATPase is increased in hypokalemia, hypokalemia exacerbates or induces digoxin toxicity**—it is wise to give pts on digoxin either a potassium-sparing diuretic, an ACE inhibitor, or both to prevent hypokalemia

    (e) Digoxin is renally cleared, thus renal failure dramatically prolongs digoxin half-life, leading to dangerous accumulation—digoxin should be avoided or dosed by close monitoring of serum levels in pts with renal failure

    (f) **Acute, severe toxicity can be reversed by Digibind, an antidigoxin antibody that serves as an antidote for digoxin**

C. Milrinone and amrinone (see Table 8.3)
1. Phosphodiesterase inhibitors $\rightarrow$ $\uparrow$ cAMP inside cells $\rightarrow$ $\uparrow$ muscle contraction, $\uparrow$ HR
2. **Unlike digoxin, leads to marked increase in myocardial O_2 consumption**
3. Useful only acutely as an IV pressor for cardiogenic shock

D. Dopamine (see Tables 8.3 & 2.8)
1. Binds to α_1-receptors in periphery and β_1-receptors on heart $\rightarrow$ $\uparrow$ cAMP inside cells
2. Causes $\uparrow$ SVR, $\uparrow$ HR, $\uparrow$ contractility $\rightarrow$ $\uparrow$ O_2 consumption
3. **Because of its effects on SVR, dopamine is most useful for hypotension caused by low SVR** (e.g., sepsis, systemic vasodilation $2°$ to other medications like dobutamine)
4. Can be used for cardiogenic shock, typically in combination with dobutamine
5. At low doses (e.g., <5 µg/kg/min) dopamine preferentially binds to special dopamine receptors in the renal vasculature, causing renal vasodilation and $\uparrow$ renal perfusion

E. Dobutamine (see Tables 8.3 & 2.8)
1. Binds to β_1-receptors on heart without having α_1 effects on periphery

2. ↑ contractility → ↑ cardiac output → autonomic reflex ↓ SVR

3. Therefore does not increase afterload, and its increase in myocardial oxygen consumption is less than dopamine's

4. **1st-line agent for acute severe heart failure**

5. **However, because of its potential to worsen hypotension, it cannot be used by itself in cardiogenic shock (e.g., in heart failure associated with refractory hypotension)**

6. It can be combined with other vasoconstrictors (usually dopamine) to reverse its induction of reflex ↓ SVR

F. Epinephrine (see Tables 8.3 & 2.8)

1. Binds to all adrenergic receptors ($\alpha_1\alpha_2\beta_1\beta_2$)

2. Most commonly used as a pressor during cardiac arrest, when given in single-doses IV push

3. Can be used as a drip when other measures are failing in cardiogenic shock

4. Causes marked increase in myocardial O_2 consumption

G. Norepinephrine (see Tables 8.3 & 2.8)

1. Although does have ⊕ inotropic effect due to β_1 agonism, its predominant effect is ↑ SVR via much more potent α_1 agonism in vasculature

2. **Therefore not very useful as an inotrope, more useful as a pressor in pts with hypotension due to ↓ SVR (e.g., sepsis)**

3. Causes a marked increase in myocardial O_2 consumption

IV. Antiarrhythmics (see Table 8.4)

A. Class I antiarrhythmics

1. Sodium channel antagonists → ↓ upstroke and amplitude of cardiac action potential → ↓ conduction velocity in injured tissues

2. Decreases pacemaker rate (especially ectopics), decreases conduction, decreases excitability

3. **Prolonged action potential → prolonged QT segment on EKG**

4. Prolonged action potential duration with ↓ conduction velocity → ↓ recovery time for conducting tissues → ↑ **risk for reentrant arrhythmias**

5. Class IA

(a) Quinidine

(1) Effective for both atrial and ventricular arrhythmias

(2) Has anticholinergic activity → ↑ AV node conduction, so may paradoxically ↑ HR by ↑ ventricular response

Table 8.4 Antiarrhythmics

Drug	Class	Characteristics
quinidine	IA	• Can be used for atrial and ventricular tachycardias • Has anticholinergic activity, can cause QT prolongation → syncope from torsade de pointes • Can induce digoxin toxicity by increasing serum levels of digoxin
procainamide	IA	• Convert wide-complex tachycardia (ventricular or supraventricular) • IV loading is limited by hypotension • Beware of drug-induced lupus and QT prolongation
disopyramide	IA	• Rarely used due to negative inotropic effects
lidocaine	IB	• Useful for treatment of refractory ventricular tachycardia or fibrillation (no longer 1st line in ACLS*), or for maintenance of normal sinus rhythm in those at risk for ventricular tachycardia (e.g., post-MI, ischemic pts) • Avoid in high-grade heart block
phenytoin	IB	• Rarely used as an antiarrhythmic
flecainide	IC	• Suppresses ventricular ectopy, but rarely used because people who take it may have increased risk of death (it is also proarrhythmic)
β-blockers	II	• 1st line for tachyarrhythmias associated with ischemia or increased sympathetic tone (e.g., hyperthyroid, etc.)
bretylium	III	• Formerly 2nd line for pulseless ventricular tachycardia/fibrillation, but completely off the ACLS algorithm, rarely used
sotalol	III	• Has β-blocking effects, most useful for atrial fibrillation cardioversion or for maintenance to keep pt out of atrial fibrillation
amiodarone	III	• 1st line for many arrhythmias, both ventricular and supraventricular • 1st line for pulseless ventricular tachycardia/fibrillation* • Beware of pulmonary fibrosis and hyperthyroidism or hypothyroidism

Table 8.4 (Continued)

Drug	Class	Characteristics
ibutilide	III	• Useful for conversion atrial fibrillation • Can induce ventricular tachycardia in pt with low ejection fraction
dofetilide	III	• Used for refractory atrial fibrillation • Associated with torsades de pointes due to its selective potassium channel blockade, resulting in QT prolongation • QT prolongation is dose related, so the drug must be administered in the hospital, and the hospital must be certified for the drug's use
verapamil, diltiazem	IV	• Useful to slow ventricular rate in atrial fibrillation • Avoid in pts with low ejection fractions or those taking β-blockers
adenosine	Misc.	• 1st line for supraventricular tachycardia, converts > 90% of them • Extremely short-acting
magnesium	Misc.	• 1st line for QT prolongation, especially torsade de pointes

Misc. = miscellaneous
*The Emergency Cardiovascular Care guidelines published by the American Heart Association list amiodarone as a Class IIb indication for pulseless V-fib/V-tach, meaning that its use is supported by "fair to good" evidence, whereas use of lidocaine is Class III, or "indeterminate," meaning that data do not exist either in support of or against its use (Circulation 2000;102:I1–11). Amiodarone has been studied in a prospective, randomized trial of out-of-hospital V-fib arrest (New Eng J Med 1999;341:871), whereas lidocaine did not improve outcomes in out-of-hospital V-fib arrest in a randomized trial (Circulation 1990;82:2027) and there are NO prospective, randomized data showing that lidocaine improves outcome in V-fib arrests. As well, amiodarone has proven effective as therapy for tachyarrhythmias that are refractory to lidocaine (J Am College Cardiol 1996;27:67). Finally, in a double-blinded, randomized, placebo-controlled head-to-head comparison of amiodarone versus lidocaine for out-of-hospital V-fib arrest, amiodarone almost doubled the rate of survival to hospital admission compared to lidocaine (N Eng J Med 2002;346:884).

to atrial fibrillation or flutter—this can be prevented by pretreatment with low doses of digoxin (cholinomimetic activity on AV node)

(3) Increases digoxin levels by inhibiting renal elimination so can induce digoxin toxicity

(4) At high doses can cause complete AV block

(5) Toxicity = hypotension (α_1 blockade), headaches, tinnitus, heart block, ventricular tachycardia, syncope (may

be caused by torsade de pointes, a form of ventricular tachycardia seen when the QT segment is prolonged)

(b) Procainamide

   (1) Useful for both ventricular tachycardia and supraventricular tachycardia

   (2) Causes hypotension via ganglionic blockade, so cannot be used in those with low BP

   (3) Metabolized in liver to N-acetylprocainamide (NAPA), which has antiarrhythmic properties and a long half-life

   (4) Procainamide and NAPA levels must be carefully monitored in renal failure due to risk of accumulation

   (5) **Can cause drug-induced lupus, hypotension (from ganglionic blockade), hepatitis, skin rash, QT prolongation**

(c) Disopyramide

   (1) Similar to quinidine but anticholinergic properties more striking

   (2) Rarely used clinically due to negative inotropic effects

6. Class IB

(a) Act on sodium channels in the ventricle with minimal effects on nodal or conducting tissue

(b) Actually shorten action potential duration (opposite of Class IA) → prolonged diastole → ↑ recovery time → ↓ **risk of reentrant arrhythmia**

(c) **These drugs have few effects in healthy cardiac tissue and mediate most of their effects in ischemic/injured tissues, so major effect is in suppressing arrhythmias associated with depolarization (e.g., ischemia, digoxin toxicity) and have minimal effects against arrhythmias in normally polarized tissues (e.g., atrial fibrillation)**

(d) Lidocaine

   (1) **Useful for stable ventricular tachycardia, can convert rhythm to normal and maintain normal rhythm in ischemic tissues**

   (2) **Previously 1st line for ventricular tachycardia/ fibrillation without a pulse (code blue), but ACLS guidelines now indicate that amiodarone is preferred (see footnote at bottom of Table 8.4)**

   (3) Must be given IV because of extensive first-pass metabolism

   (4) Toxicity is primarily CNS → seizures, drowsiness, paresthesias

(5) **Should not be used in high-grade heart block, because it suppresses ventricular automaticity and therefore may prevent a ventricular escape rhythm, which may be necessary to keep alive a pt with complete block**

(e) Phenytoin

(1) Rarely used as an antiarrhythmic, typically used as an antiseizure medicine (see Tables 3.11 & 3.12)

(2) Effects are similar to lidocaine, but less marked

7. Class IC

(a) Markedly slow conduction velocity by slowing initial depolarization, used principally for ventricular arrhythmias

(b) Extremely effective at suppressing premature ventricular contractions and at slowing the ventricular response to atrial flutter or fibrillation

(c) Rarely used due to their proarrhythmogenic effects, may ↑ risk of death

(d) Flecainide is the major drug in the class

B. Class II drugs

1. **These are β-blockers, specifically β₁ antagonists**

2. **1st-line antiarrhythmics for most conditions because they actually improve survival, unlike most other agents**

3. Particularly useful for ischemic pts, or tachycardias due to increased sympathetic state, but also very useful to rate control atrial fibrillation/flutter

C. Class III drugs

1. A grab-bag class of drugs, each with mixed and varying actions

2. They all share one common property: they prolong the action potential duration without altering initial depolarization or the resting membrane potential

3. **Thus, these drugs increase the strength of an electrical stimulus needed to induce ventricular fibrillation**

4. **Their principal use is intractable ventricular tachycardia/ fibrillation**

5. Bretylium

(a) Previously a 2nd-line agent for pulseless ventricular tachycardia or fibrillation (code blue), but now has been completely removed from the ACLS protocol

(b) Tended to cause severe vomiting, worldwide supplies are limited, and drug had limited efficacy in code blue setting

6. Sotalol
   (a) An interesting class III agent that **ALSO is a β-blocker**
   (b) **Useful to convert atrial fibrillation/flutter, either alone or as a sensitizer to electrical cardioversion**
   (c) Also useful to prevent ventricular tachyarrhythmias, typically used over the long term rather than in acute/emergent situations
7. Amiodarone
   (a) Has become the darling drug of the ACLS protocols, indicated 1st or 2nd line for virtually every arrhythmia
   (b) **Most importantly is now considered 1st line for refractory pulseless ventricular tachycardia or fibrillation (see footnote at bottom of Table 8.4)**
   (c) **Also a 1st-line agent for supraventricular tachycardias**
   (d) Can be used acutely or chronically
   (e) Toxicity is profound
      (1) **Pulmonary fibrosis is irreversible and may be dose-related (loosely), but it can occur at any time during therapy**
      (2) **Amiodarone contains iodine and can cause either hyperthyroid or hypothyroid**
      (3) Can also cause hepatic necrosis/fibrosis
   (f) Amiodarone accumulates in fatty tissues and has an elimination half-life of three months
8. Ibutilide
   (a) **Principal use is for atrial fibrillation**, can convert to sinus by itself, and also markedly improves efficacy of electrical cardioversion
   (b) In patients with low ejection fractions it can induce ventricular tachycardia
9. Dofetilide
   (a) Highly effective at converting refractory atrial fibrillation
   (b) However, due to its selective inhibition of potassium channels, the drug causes dose-related QT prolongation, and is associated with torsades de pointes
   (c) As a result, the FDA has mandated that any patient receiving this drug must be hospitalized for 72 hours in a monitored setting, and only hospitals certified to have been trained in the drug's use by the manufacturer are allowed to administer it

D. Class IV agents
  1. Calcium channel blockers—nondihydropyridines
  2. Predominant effect is on the SA and AV nodes
  3. **Can abort reentrant tachycardias and can slow ventricular rate in atrial fibrillation/flutter**
  4. Major adverse effect is negative inotropic actions, which can lead to worsening heart failure
  5. Also should not be combined with class II agents (β-blockers) because of risk of induction of complete heart block

E. Miscellaneous
  1. Adenosine
    (a) **Binds to adenosine receptors in AV node → marked, immediate ↓ in AV node conduction**
    (b) **1st-line agent for supraventricular tachycardias**
    (c) **Causes immediate cessation of AV nodal reentrant tachycardias, restoring sinus rhythm in > 90% of cases**
    (d) Also useful as a diagnostic maneuver in wide complex tachycardias of unknown origin—if it is supraventricular it will terminate, if it is ventricular it won't
    (e) It causes marked flushing and chest burning, very uncomfortable for the pt, and also may induce high-grade heart block, very uncomfortable for the physician watching the rhythm on the monitor as he/she is pushing the drug!
    (f) Fortunately has an extremely short half-life (a few seconds), so effects wear off in < 10 seconds
  2. Magnesium
    (a) 1st-line agent for torsade de pointes, typically seen in conditions with QT prolongation
    (b) Magnesium shortens the QT duration

9. HEMATOLOGIC AGENTS

I. Anticoagulants (see Table 9.1)

A. Unfractionated heparin

1. Mixture of mucopolysaccharides of varying size, weight, and shape
2. Catalytically accelerates by 1000-fold the interaction of antithrombin III and thrombin, thereby inactivating thrombin
3. **Given subcutaneously for prophylaxis of deep vein thrombosis (DVT), given by IV drip for therapy for deep vein thrombosis or pulmonary embolus**
4. **Highly unreliable bioavailability means serum levels must be followed by checking the partial thromboplastin time (PTT)**
5. Adverse effects are uncontrolled hemorrhage and induction of **heparin-induced thrombocytopenia**, an autoimmune phenomenon in which heparin acts as an adjuvant by binding to platelet factor 4, thereby inducing antibodies that bind platelets, **leading to a paradoxical hypercoagulable state**
6. Heparin should not be used in a patient who is actively bleeding, who has a serious bleeding diathesis, or who has a history of heparin-induced thrombocytopenia
7. **Protamine sulfate is a heparin antidote, which can rapidly reverse heparin if a patient develops bleeding**

Table 9.1 Anticoagulants, Thrombolytics, & Procoagulants

Drug	Characteristics
heparin (unfractionated)	• Unreliable bioavailability, IV drip must be monitored by following the PTT
	• Used subcutaneously for DVT prophylaxis, IV for therapy of DVT
	• Rapidly reversible with protamine sulfate
LMWH	• Much more reliable bioavailability, and specific inhibition of Factor X
	• Used subcutaneously for DVT prophylaxis or therapy

Table 9.1 (Continued)

Drug	Characteristics
gpIIbIIIa antagonists	• Eptifibatide, abciximab (ReoPro), and tirofiban are the drugs available • Used in conjunction with unfractionated heparin drip for patients with unstable angina, non–ST-elevation myocardial infarction, or those receiving angioplasty
lepirudin bivalirudin	• Both based on leech saliva; lepirudin, a purified component; and bivalirudin, a synthetic peptide • Both are direct thrombin inhibitors (work independent of antithrombin III) indicated for patients with heparin-induced thrombocytopenia
fondaparinux	• A nonheparin anticoagulant, selective antithrombin-III mediated inhibitor of Factor Xa • Indicated for DVT prophylaxis, especially in patients with heparin-induced thrombocytopenia, major risk is bleeding or thrombocytopenia (both rare) • Advantages over other nonheparin anticoagulants (e.g. lepirudin & argatroban) are the once daily SQ dosing and lack of need for continuous infusion or monitoring
argatroban	• Direct thrombin inhibitor that works independently of antithrombin III (in contrast to heparin & fondaparinux) • Indicated for patients with heparin-induced thrombocytopenia, derivative of L-arginine
coumadin	• The most effective oral anticoagulant, used for outpatient therapy of DVT, atrial fibrillation, or other severe hypercoagulable state
aspirin	• Used to prevent stroke and myocardial infarction, 2nd-line agent for atrial fibrillation
ticlopidine	• Added to aspirin if stroke develops while on aspirin therapy; also used if stents are placed during angioplasty • Risk of TTP has diminished its use in recent years
clopidogrel	• Same uses as ticlopidine, but appears to be safer, lower risk of TTP

(Continued)

Table 9.1 (Continued)

Drug	Characteristics
dipyridamole (Persantine)	• Weakly prevents platelet aggregation, rarely used for this • Vasodilator useful for cardiac stress tests
drotrecogin alpha	• Recombinant activated protein C, inhibits intravascular coagulation • Proven to decrease mortality in severe sepsis, can cause bleeding
tPA	• Recombinant analog of the body's natural activator of plasmin • Only activates plasmin in the immediate vicinity of a formed fibrin clot • 1st-line Tx for myocardial infarction (within 12 hrs of Sx onset, preferably within 90 min) & ischemic stroke (within 3 hrs of Sx onset)
streptokinase	• Nonspecific activator of plasmin, causing fibrinolysis • Indicated for myocardial infarction (within 12 hrs, 90 min preferred)
urokinase	• Nonspecific activator of plasmin, causing fibrinolysis • Indicated for myocardial infarction (within 12 hrs, 90 min preferred)
aminocaproic acid	• Inhibits fibrinolysis by antagonizing plasmin • Reverses thrombolytic therapy
tranexamic acid	• Inhibits fibrinolysis by antagonizing plasmin • Reverses thrombolytic therapy
protamine sulfate	• Reverses unfractionated heparin
desmopressin	• Assists clotting by causing von Willebrand's factor release • Specifically used to correct bleeding caused by dysfunctional platelets (especially Type I von Willebrand's Dz, hemophilia, uremia)
Advate	• Recombinant human Factor VIII, administered to hemophiliacs to reduce bleeding

B. Low molecular weight heparin (LMWH)

1. **Purification of the active heparin polymers and elimination of larger, less active polymers means that LMWH has much more reliable bioavailability**

2. **In addition, LMWH is far more specific at inhibiting Factor X than is unfractionated heparin**

3. **Thus LMWH can be administered subcutaneously, and serum assays of anticoagulation do not need to be followed**

4. These drugs have been proven to be as effective as unfractionated heparin in a variety of settings, including deep vein thrombosis prevention and treatment

5. Bleeding risk is somewhat lower with LMWH, as is the risk of initiating heparin-induced thrombocytopenia—**however, LMWH will cross-react in a patient who already has heparin-induced thrombocytopenia, so LMWH cannot be used in these patients, and a non-heparin-based anticoagulant must be used**

6. However, if a patient has an underlying bleeding diathesis or is at high risk for bleeding (e.g., recent surgery), unfractionated heparin drip is preferred not only because it can be reversed with protamine and LMWH cannot, but also because the body clears unfractionated heparin within a matter of hours when the drip is turned off, whereas LWMH administered subcutaneously continues to be absorbed for at least12 hours

C. gpIIbIIIa antagonists

1. The gpIIbIIIa receptor on platelets binds to von Willebrand's factor, thereby bridging platelets to a fibrin clot and to the subendothelial matrix

2. **Antagonists of the gpIIbIIIa receptor (based on venom from cobras) have been shown to reduce the cumulative risk of death, recurrent myocardial infarction, or recurrent unstable angina in patients with unstable angina or non-ST-elevation myocardial infarction**

3. In addition, these agents have been shown to reduce the risk of stent reocclusion following angioplasty of a narrowed coronary artery

4. They are administered by continuous IV drip in combination with unfractionated heparin drip

5. They do increase the risk of severe hemorrhage, and unlike unfractionated heparin, cannot be rapidly reversed

D. Nonheparin parenteral anticoagulants
1. Lepirudin & Bivalirudin
   (a) Lepirudin is a derivative of leech saliva, and bivalirudin is a synthetic peptide based on proteins in leech saliva
   (b) Both are direct thrombin inhibitors (do not require antithrombin III for effect)
   (c) Safe to use in patients with heparin-induced thrombocytopenia
   (d) However, the drugs must be dosed by continuous infusion, and anticoagulant effect requires monitoring
   (e) Anaphylaxis can occur
2. Fondaparinux
   (a) A synthetic pentasaccharide structure based on the structure of heparin, but it specifically interacts with Factor X (via antithrombin III)
   (b) Convenient once daily SQ dosing, and no monitoring is required
   (c) An option for therapy in patients with heparin-induced thrombocytopenia
3. Argatroban
   (a) A small molecule based on the structure of L-arginine, it works as a direct thrombin inhibitor, not requiring antithrombin III
   (b) Indicated for patients with heparin-induced thrombocytopenia
   (c) Dosed IV, in contrast to fondaparinux
E. Coumadin
1. **The only currently available oral anticoagulant that is as effective as heparin**
2. **Coumadin antagonizes the vitamin K–dependent gamma carboxylation of the terminal glutamate residues of Factors II, VII, IX, and X by gamma glutamate carboxylase** (see Figure 9.1)
3. Gamma glutamate carboxylation is necessary to provide the factors with the negative charge needed to interact with the divalent cation calcium during clot formation
4. Coumadin is cumbersome to dose and monitor, requiring regular blood draws to check the level of anticoagulation by assessing the prothrombin time (PT)
5. It typically takes 3–5 days for the full therapeutic effect of coumadin to occur because of the long half-life of the affected factors

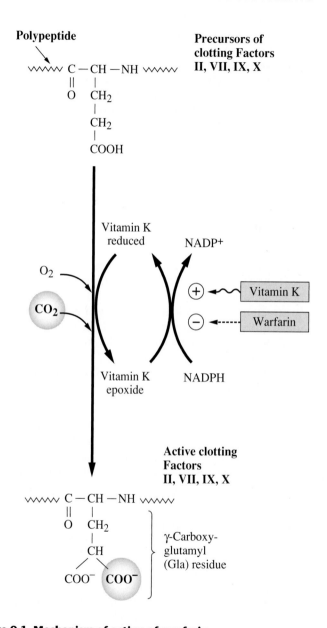

Figure 9.1 Mechanism of action of warfarin
(Redrawn from Howland RD, Mycek MJ, Harvey RA, Champe PC. Lippincott's Illustrated Reviews: Pharmacology, 2nd ed. Baltimore: Lippincott Williams & Wilkins, 2001:200.)

6. Because protein C and protein S, which are antithrombotic circulating proteins, are also affected by gamma glutamate carboxylase, and because these proteins have a shorter half-life than Factors II, VII, IX, and X, coumadin may cause a temporary HYPERcoagulable state when first started—this can cause the infamous "warfarin-induced skin necrosis," which is caused by thromboemboli lodging in peripheral cutaneous capillaries

7. For this reason, heparin drip is often started before coumadin therapy is begun, and heparin is continued until the PT is therapeutic—warfarin-induced skin necrosis is quite rare and probably only occurs in patients with some underlying hypercoagulable state, so the need for heparin drip is some-what controversial in most patients

F. Aspirin

1. Acts via inhibition of formation of platelet thromboxane (see Figure 9.2) , preventing platelet aggregation, thereby increasing bleeding time

2. **An effective anticoagulant, it serves as a 2nd-line oral anticoagulant for patients with atrial fibrillation and should be given to ALL patients with risks for, or a history of, myocardial infarction or stroke**

3. Should be given to all patients with chest pain as soon as they present to the emergency room

G. Ticlopidine

1. Acts via inhibition of ADP activation of platelet aggregation

2. More potent than aspirin, and previously added to aspirin when strokes occurred in the face of aspirin therapy; however, it has been associated with cases of thrombotic thrombocytopenic purpura (TTP) and is now being replaced by clopidogrel

H. Clopidogrel

1. **Works similarly to ticlopidine, but seems to be safer—although recent case reports have also described TTP with clopidogrel therapy** (see Figure 9.3)

2. Should be added to patients who develop strokes on aspirin, used for myocardial infarction and stroke prophylaxis in pa-tients who cannot tolerate aspirin, and used for all patients who receive stents during angioplasty

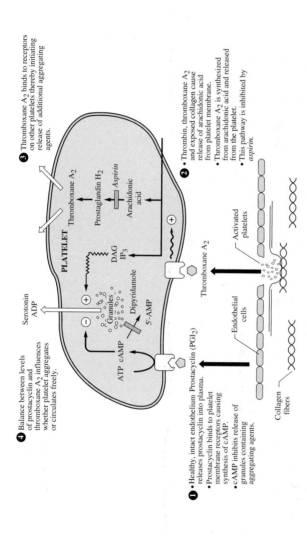

Figure 9.2 Chemical mediators influencing platelet activation and aggregation (relative size of platelets and endothelial cells are not to scale)

(Redrawn from Howland RD, Mycek MJ, Harvey RA, Champe PC. Lippincott's Illustrated Reviews: Pharmacology, 2nd ed. Baltimore: Lippincott Williams & Wilkins, 2001:195.)

❶ • Healthy, intact endothelium releases prostacyclin into plasma.
• Prostacyclin binds to platelet membrane receptors causing synthesis of cAMP.
• cAMP inhibits release of granules containing aggregating agents.

❷ • Thrombin, thromboxane A₂ and exposed collagen cause release of arachidonic acid from platelet membrane.
• Thromboxane A₂ is synthesized from arachidonic acid and released from the platelet.
• This pathway is inhibited by *aspirin*.

❸ Thromboxane A₂ binds to receptors on other platelets thereby initiating release of additional aggregating agents.

❹ Balance between levels of prostacyclin and thromboxane A₂ influences whether platelet aggregates or circulates freely.

PLATELET

Thromboxane A₂

Prostaglandin H₂

Aspirin

Arachidonic acid

Serotonin
ADP

Granules

DAG
IP₃

Dipyridamole

ATP cAMP

5'-AMP

Prostacyclin (PGI₂)

Thromboxane A₂

Endothelial cells

Activated platelets

Collagen fibers

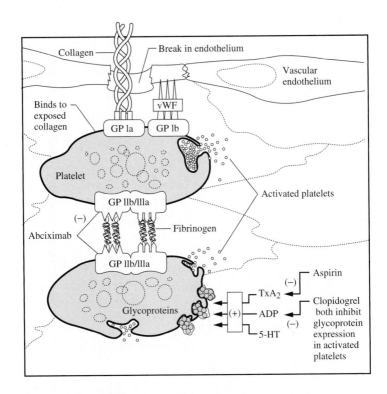

Figure 9.3 Mechanism of antiplatelet action
(Redrawn from Bhushan V, Le, T. First Aid for the USMLE Step 1:2005. New York: McGraw-Hill, 2005:325. Adapted with permission from Katzung BG, Trevor AJ. USMLE Road Map: Pharmacology, 1st ed. New York: McGraw-Hill: 56.)

I. Dipyridamole (Persantine)

1. Weakly decreases platelet aggregation

2. Also acts as a vasodilator, and so is used in cardiac stress tests when the pt cannot exercise (e.g., from disabling arthritis, etc.), works by vasodilating coronaries, except diseased coronaries do not vasodilate well, so dipyridamole induces a "steal" phenomenon in which diseased coronaries get less blood flow, thereby inducing local ischemia

3. Persantine also causes reflex tachycardia due to vasodilation, thereby increasing the myocardial oxygen demand

4. Rarely used as an antiplatelet drug

J. Drotrecogin alpha (recombinant activated protein C)
   1. The first ever biological therapy proven effective for treatment of sepsis
   2. Inhibits intravascular coagulation, leading to improved survival in severe sepsis

II. Thrombolytics (see Table 9.1)

A. "Clot-busters," the three in use are tissue plasminogen activator (tPA), streptokinase, and urokinase
B. **tPA is a recombinant activator of plasmin, but it only activates plasmin locally in the area of a fibrin-containing clot, making it a "fibrin-specific clot-buster"**
C. **Streptokinase and urokinase activate the promolecule plasminogen,** converting it into its active form plasmin, which degrades fibrin all over the body, even that contained in the promolecule fibrinogen
D. All three have been proven to reduce the risk of death when administered to patients with myocardial infarction within 12 hours of onset of symptoms—there is a steady decrease in efficacy as time passes, so the goal is a "door-to-drug time" of 90 min or less, although up to 6 hours results are very beneficial, whereas up to 12 hours the benefit becomes marginal
E. tPA may be slightly more effective/safe
F. **tPA also proven to improve survival and neurologic outcome in patients with nonhemorrhagic strokes if given within 3 hours of onset of symptoms**
G. All three have risks for causing severe hemorrhage, but streptokinase and urokinase may also cause hypersensitivity/anaphylactoid reactions

III. Procoagulants (see Table 9.1)

A. Aminocaproic acid & tranexamic acid
   1. **Inhibit fibrinolysis by antagonizing plasmin**
   2. Useful to reverse thrombolytic therapy, or to treat any uncontrolled bleeding
B. Protamine sulfate reverses the effects of heparin, acting as a rapid antidote in case hemorrhage develops while on heparin therapy
C. Desmopressin (DDAVP)
   1. **Used to stimulate release of von Willebrand's factor from endothelial cells →↑ clotting**

2. Tachyphylaxis develops after 1–2 doses because of depletion of preformed von Willebrand's factor from the endothelium, and 24–48 hours is necessary to allow synthesis of new factor
3. Can be administered by nasal spray, subcutaneously, or IV
4. Most effective for bleeding due to von Willebrand's disease (especially Type I, contraindicated in Type II) or hemophilia, but can also help in uremia or other conditions associated with dysfunctional platelets
5. Causes hyponatremia as a side effect

IV. Hematopoietic Agents (see Table 9.2)

A. Recombinant erythropoietin

1. **Erythropoietin is the major hormone responsible for red blood cell production, normally produced in the kidney**
2. The recombinant version is used in patients with renal failure, increases hematocrit toward normal

Table 9.2 Hematopoietic Agents

Drug	Characteristics
erythropoietin darbepoetin	• Recombinant human erythropoietin stimulates red blood cell production • Darbepoetin is a highly glycosylated erythropoietin molecule with a longer half-life, allowing once weekly dosing • Stimulates red blood cell production, used to increase hematocrit in patients with renal failure (low EPO state) or chemotherapy-related anemia
filgrastim PEG-filgrastim	• Filgrastim is recombinant human granulocyte-colony stimulating factor (G-CSF), which stimulates neutrophil production • PEG = polyethylene glycol, the addition of which to filgrastim markedly prolongs circulating half-life and increases effect • Chiefly used to increase neutrophil recovery after chemotherapy
anagrelide	• Inhibits platelet formation, used for any pt with high platelets
oprelvekin	• Recombinant human interleukin-11 • Stimulates platelet production after chemotherapy

3. Also used by athletes to dope their blood ($\uparrow$ hematocrit $\rightarrow \uparrow O_2$ carrying capacity)

4. Can be administered subcutaneously or intravenously

5. Minimal side effects

B. Filgrastim [recombinant granulocyte-colony stimulating factor (G-CSF)]

1. **G-CSF is a key hormone in stimulating neutrophil formation**

2. Name comes from: neutrophil (**fil**), **gra**nulocyte, **stim**ulator = fil-gra-stim

3. G-CSF is used to increase white blood cell counts in patients receiving chemotherapy or who have other conditions associated with neutropenia (e.g., AIDS)

4. Can also be used to mobilize bone marrow stem cells into the peripheral blood for harvesting of the stem cells prior to bone marrow transplant

5. Can be administered subcutaneously or intravenously

6. Can cause diffuse bone pain as hematopoiesis is stimulated all over the body

C. Anagrelide

1. Inhibits formation of platelets from mature megakaryocytes

2. Mechanism of action unknown

3. Used for conditions of thrombocytosis, either for essential thrombocythemia or for any reactive cause

4. Causes caffeine-like effects, including headaches, tremor, anxiety, nausea

10. CHEMOTHERAPY

I. Alkylating Agents

A. General characteristics (see Table 10.1)

1. All alkylating agents are reactive compounds that damage DNA and/or proteins in the cell, thereby inhibiting cell replication

2. Note that if the cells are not killed outright, then mutations will be induced—**thus, alkylating agents are mutagenic, therefore carcinogenic (they induce secondary cancers)**

3. Toxicity

(a) Many alkylating agents are strong vesicants, meaning they cause tissue necrosis if leaked into tissues around the IV site (e.g., due to a faulty IV)

(b) Nausea/vomiting occur within hours of infusion

(c) Dose-related sloughing of GI tract lining, alopecia, and sterility

(d) **Bone marrow suppression is the major dose-limiting toxicity** and typically involves the neutrophils and platelets more than red cells (which have a longer half-life)

4. Resistance to alkylating agents can be due to upregulation of DNA repair mechanisms, decreased penetration of the drug into the malignant cell, or increased production of glutathione, which neutralizes alkylating agents

B. Mechlorethamine, melphalan, chlorambucil, busulfan (see Table 10.2)

1. All four drugs are used mostly for hematologic malignancies

(a) Mechlorethamine is part of the MOPP regimen for Hodgkin's disease: MOPP = mechlorethamine, Oncovin (vincristine), procarbazine, prednisone

(b) Melphalan combined with prednisone is one of the common therapies for multiple myeloma

(c) Chlorambucil and busulfan are used in leukemias or lymphoma

(d) **Busulfan causes pulmonary fibrosis** (along with bleomycin, the "killer B" drugs)

C. Cyclophosphamide

1. Unlike other alkylating agents, cyclophosphamide is NOT a vesicant

Table 10.1 Chemotherapy Class Toxicities

Class of Drugs	Characteristics
classic alkylating agents	• Vesicants (tissue necrosis), nausea/vomiting, alopecia, & sterility • Dose-limiting toxicity is bone marrow suppression • All are carcinogenic, that is, they induce secondary cancers
nitrosoureas[a]	• Cross the blood-brain barrier so useful for CNS cancers
platinum agents[a]	• Useful for testicular, ovarian, and germ cell tumors • Cisplatin (but not carboplatin) causes milder bone marrow suppression than other agents • Ototoxicity, peripheral neuropathy, and renal failure are 1° problems
antibiotics	• Variable indications and toxicities, typically cause bone marrow toxicity • Bleomycin causes pulmonary fibrosis
anthracyclines[b]	• Cause dose-related cardiac toxicity, very broad-spectrum activity
antimetabolites	• Variable indications and toxicities
purine antagonists[c]	• Useful for leukemias, cause bone marrow toxicity
pyrimidine antagonists[c]	• Useful for GI adenocarcinomas, cause bone marrow toxicity
vinca alkaloids	• Used for leukemia, cause peripheral neuropathy (more for vincristine)
podophyllotoxins	• Used for lung and testicular cancer, cause bone marrow toxicity
taxanes	• Used for breast and ovarian cancer, cause bone marrow toxicity
endocrine	• Hormone therapies for breast and prostate cancer, steroids for lymphoma, side effects are mild
biological modifiers	• Variable, toxicity mild for antibodies, more severe for cytokines

[a]Nitrosoureas and platinum agents are subclasses of alkylating agents.
[b]Anthracycline is a subclass of antibiotic.
[c]Purine and pyrimidine antagonists are subclasses of antimetabolites.

CHEMOTHERAPY

Table 10.2 Chemotherapy Agents

Drug	Class	Clinical Uses	Major Toxicity
mechlorethamine	Alkylating agent	Lymphoma	Bone marrow: induce 2° cancer
melphalan	Alkylating agent	Multiple myeloma	Bone marrow: induce 2° cancer
chlorambucil	Alkylating agent	Leukemia/lymphoma	Bone marrow: induce 2° cancer
busulfan	Alkylating agent	Leukemia/lymphoma	Lung fibrosis: induce 2° cancer
cyclophosphamide	Alkylating agent	Leukemia/lymphoma/breast	Bone marrow: hemorrhagic cystitis: induce 2° cancer
ifosfamide	Alkylating agent	Testicular/sarcomas	Bone marrow: hemorrhagic cystitis: induce 2° cancer
thiotepa	Alkylating agent	Ovarian	Bone marrow: induce 2° cancer
temozolomide	Alkylating agent	CNS tumor	Bone marrow
dacarbazine	Alkylating agent	Lymphoma	Bone marrow: induce 2° cancer
procarbazine	Alkylating agent	Lymphoma	Bone marrow: induce 2° cancer
carmustine	Nitrosoureas[a]	CNS tumor	Bone marrow: vomiting
lomustine	Nitrosoureas[a]	CNS tumor	Bone marrow: vomiting
cisplatin	Platinum[a]	Head & neck/germ cell	Ototoxicity: neuropathy: renal

Table 10.2 (Continued)

Drug	Class	Clinical Uses	Major Toxicity
carboplatin	Platinum[a]	Ovarian/lung	As cisplatin, but much milder
oxaliplatin	Platinum[a]	Colon	Neuropathy, worse when cold
doxorubicin	Anthracycline[b]	Broad spectrum	Cardiac toxicity
daunorubicin	Anthracycline[b]	Leukemia	Cardiac toxicity
idarubicin	Anthracycline[b]	Leukemia	Cardiac toxicity
dactinomycin	Antibiotic	Wilms' tumor	Bone marrow
plicamycin	Antibiotic	Hypercalcemia	Bone marrow
mitomycin	Antibiotic	Cervical/GI	Bone marrow
bleomycin	Antibiotic	GU/lymphoma	Lung fibrosis: anaphylaxis
irinotecan	Antibiotic	Colon	Bone marrow: diarrhea
methotrexate	Antimetabolite	Leukemia/breast	Bone marrow: GI: liver fibrosis
pemetrexed	Antimetabolite	Mesothelioma	Bone marrow
mercaptopurine	Purine analog[c]	Leukemia	Bone marrow
thioguanine	Purine analog[c]	Leukemia	Bone marrow
fludarabine	Purine analog[c]	Leukemia	Bone marrow
hydroxyurea	Purine analog[c]	Lymphoproliferative	Bone marrow
cladribine	Purine analog[c]	Leukemia	Bone marrow
5-fluorouracil	Pyrimidine analog[c]	GI adenocarcinoma	Bone marrow
capecitabine	Pyrimidine analog[c]	GI adenocarcinoma	Bone marrow
gemcitabine	Pyrimidine analog[c]	GI adenocarcinoma	Bone marrow
cytarabine	Pyrimidine analog[c]	Leukemia	Bone marrow
azacytidine	Pyrimidine analog[c]	Myelodysplastic syndrome	Bone marrow, allergic
bortezomib	Proteosome inhibitor	Multiple myeloma	Bone marrow, GI
vincristine	Vinca alkaloids	Leukemia/lymphoma	Peripheral
vinblastine	Vinca alkaloids	Germ cell/lymphoma	Bone marrow

(*Continued*)

Table 10.2 (Continued)

Drug	Class	Clinical Uses	Major Toxicity
vinorelbine	Vinca alkaloids	Breast/lung	Bone marrow
etoposide	Podophyllotoxin	Testicular/lung	Bone marrow
paclitaxel	Taxane	Breast/ovarian	Bone marrow
docetaxel	Taxane	Breast/ovarian	Bone marrow
tamoxifen	Endocrine	Breast	Hot flashes, endometrial cancer
glucocorticoids	Endocrine	Leukemia/lymphoma	Diabetes, infections
leuprolide	Endocrine	Prostate	Hot flashes
flutamide	Endocrine	Prostate	Gynecomastia
ATRA	Biological	Myeloid leukemia M_3	respiratory distress, pleural effusion, pericarditis, pneumonitis
rituximab	Biological	Lymphoma	Minimal
trastuzumab	Biological	Breast	Minimal
gemtuzumab	Biological	Myeloid leukemia	Unclear
alemtuzumab	Biological	Leukemia	Bone marrow
tositumomab	Biological	Lymphoma	Allergy
ibritumomab	Biological	Lymphoma	Allergy
bevacizumab	Biological	Colon	Cardiovascular
cetuximab	Biological	Colon	Allergy
interleukin-2	Biological	Renal cell/melanoma	Capillary leak syndrome
interferon-α	Biological	Leukemia/Kaposi's sarcoma	Flulike illness: depression
imatinib mesylate (Gleevec)	Biological	CML	Unclear

[a]Nitrosoureas, platinum, and anthracycline drugs are all subclasses of alkylating agents.

[b]Anthracycline is a subclass of antibiotics.

[c]Purine and pyrimidine antagonists are subclasses of antimetabolites.

2. **This is because it must be converted to a toxic metabolite in the liver before it can mediate chemotherapeutic effect**—conversion is by the p450 enzyme

3. Cyclophosphamide can be given orally or IV, is one of the most widely used of the chemotherapy agents

4. Cancer regimens
   (a) Part of the CHOP regimen, the most commonly used regimen for lymphoma: CHOP = cyclophosphamide, H (hydroxydaunorubicin), Oncovin (vincristine), prednisone
   (b) Part of the CAF or CMF regimens for breast cancer: CAF = cyclophosphamide, Adriamycin, 5-fluorouracil; CMF = cyclophosphamide, methotrexate, 5-fluorouracil
   (c) Used in a variety of regimens for other cancers as well

5. Immunosuppressive regimens
   (a) Cyclophosphamide also used in autoimmune processes to induce remission
   (b) These can include steroid refractory autoimmune thrombocytopenia, lupus nephritis, and all kinds of vasculitis

6. Toxicities
   (a) Bone marrow toxicity results in cell counts that reach nadir at 10–12 days, typically resolves around day 21
   (b) **Hemorrhagic cystitis**
      (1) **Acrolein is a cyclophosphamide metabolite, which is highly toxic to the bladder**
      (2) Can cause hemorrhagic cystitis, which predisposes to bladder cancer in the future, and is prevented by aggressive fluid hydration
      (3) **Mesna is an antidote for acrolein, which is infused when high doses of cyclophosphamide are given**

D. Ifosfamide
   1. Closely related to cyclophosphamide, sharing the same major toxicities
   2. Ifosfamide is always given with mesna
   3. Used principally for testicular carcinoma and sarcomas

E. Triethylenethiophosphoramide (thiotepa) was formerly used for ovarian cancer

F. Dacarbazine, procarbazine
   1. Both can be used for lymphomas
   2. Dacarbazine must be activated by the hepatic cytochrome p450 system and is part of the ABVD regimen: ABVD = Adriamycin, bleomycin, vinblastine, dacarbazine

3. Procarbazine is part of the MOPP regimen
4. Procarbazine has a strong tendency to induce secondary tumors, and it crosses the blood-brain barrier so can cause CNS toxicity

G. Nitrosoureas (see Table 10.1)

1. The drugs in this class are carmustine (BCNU) and lomustine (CCNU)
2. These drugs are highly lipophilic and thus cross the blood-brain barrier, making them most useful for treatment of brain tumors
3. Cause bone marrow suppression and GI toxicity

H. Cisplatin, carboplatin, oxaliplatin

1. Platinum-derivative chemotherapy is most useful for genitourinary cancers, such as testicular carcinoma, germ cell tumors, and ovarian cancer, but can also be used for lung cancer
2. **Cisplatin causes only mild bone marrow toxicity, and its chief toxicity is renal failure, ototoxicity, peripheral neuropathies, and severe vomiting**
3. **Carboplatin causes much less renal failure, ototoxicity, and neuropathy, but more bone marrow suppression**
4. Oxaliplatin is a new agent that causes a unique peripheral neuropathy exacerbated by cold

I. Temozolomide

1. A newly approved drug indicated specifically for glioblastoma multiforme
2. An analogue of dacarbazine

II. Antibiotics (see Table 10.1)

A. General characteristics

1. These agents work by affecting DNA, either by intercalating between the base pairs, by mediating oxidative damage to DNA, or by inhibiting topoisomerase
2. Most of these agents are derivatives of the soil fungus *Streptomyces*

B. Anthracyclines (see Table 10.1)

1. Three drugs available: doxorubicin, daunorubicin, idarubicin
2. All cause DNA intercalation, DNA strand rupture, and oxidative damage

3. **The principal side effect of anthracyclines is cardiotoxicity, which is dose-related, causing dilated cardiomyopathy**

4. Can also cause bone marrow suppression, alopecia, nausea/vomiting, and are vesicants

5. Doxorubicin (Adriamycin)

   (a) One of the most widely used chemotherapeutic agents, broad spectrum of action

   (b) Serves as part of the CHOP regimen for lymphomas

   (c) Used in a variety of carcinomas, including breast and bladder

   (d) Also used for a range of sarcomas and leukemias

   g. Daunorubicin and idarubicin are chiefly used in leukemias and have narrower spectrum of action

C. Dactinomycin

   1. A DNA intercalator that inhibits RNA synthesis

   2. The dose-limiting toxicity is bone marrow suppression, but GI toxicity, mucositis, and alopecia also occur, and the drug is a vesicant

   3. Uses are limited: Wilms' tumor, choriocarcinoma

D. Plicamycin (also called mithramycin)

   1. Binds to DNA and inhibits RNA synthesis, and also inhibits osteoclast activity

   2. Toxicities include GI upset, bone marrow suppression, liver toxicity

   3. Has few cancer indications, formerly used for hypercalcemia but rarely is used now

E. Mitomycin

   1. Converted to an alkylating agent in the body

   2. May be used for cervical cancer or GI adenocarcinomas

   3. The major toxicity is severe bone marrow suppression, but it is also classically associated with hemolytic-uremic syndrome

F. Bleomycin

   1. Binds to and fragments DNA strands by oxidative reactions

   2. **The toxicity to remember is pulmonary fibrosis** (along with busulfan, the "killer Bs" cause pulmonary fibrosis)

   3. Can also cause anaphylaxis, but of note, it does NOT cause significant bone marrow toxicity

   4. Useful for a variety of GU cancers and lymphoma

G. Irinotecan
1. Inhibits topoisomerase I enzyme, leading to fragmentation of DNA during cell replication
2. Causes bone marrow suppression and severe diarrhea
3. Useful for advanced colon cancer and lung cancer

III. Antimetabolites (see Table 10.1)

A. General characteristics
1. Act as structural analogs of normal cellular metabolites
2. Many are prodrugs that are converted to the active form by normal cellular enzymes

B. Methotrexate
1. **Folic acid analog binds to and inhibits dihydrofolate reductase**
2. Because folate is necessary for pyrimidine synthesis, this depletes the cell of nucleotides → inhibition of DNA, RNA, and protein synthesis
3. Leucovorin rescue
   (1) Folinic acid (leucovorin) is the product of dihydrofolate reductase
   (2) **Folinic acid can be added after methotrexate administration to save slowly replicating, healthy tissues**
4. Major toxicities include bone marrow suppression and GI tract lining damage, and long-term accumulation of drug → hepatic fibrosis
5. Useful to treat leukemias and breast cancer, also collagen vascular diseases and psoriasis
6. Typically given intrathecally in childhood acute lymphoblastic leukemia (ALL) to prevent CNS relapse of the leukemia

C. Pemetrexed
1. Also inhibits dihydrofolate reductase, as well as thymidylate synthase
2. Used to treat mesothelioma

D. Purine antagonists
1. Mercaptopurine and thioguanine
   (a) 6-mercaptopurine and 6-thioguanine are metabolized inside the cell to nucleotide analogs, which prevent purine synthesis
   (b) These drugs are useful for leukemia Tx

(c) Azathioprine is an immunosuppressive agent useful for collagen vascular diseases and autoimmune diseases; it works by being converted to 6-mercaptopurine inside the cell (i.e., azathioprine is a pro-prodrug)

(d) Xanthine oxidase

(1) **Xanthine oxidase is the enzyme that converts azathioprine to 6-mercaptopurine, but also converts mercaptopurine to a harmless metabolite**

(2) **Thus xanthine oxidase inhibitor (allopurinol), which is frequently given to patients with leukemia to prevent tumor lysis syndrome, inhibits the effect of the precursor drug azathioprine, but potentiates the effects of the derivative drug, 6-mercaptopurine**

(3) Azathioprine doses must be markedly increased in the presence of xanthine oxidase, but 6-mercaptopurine doses must be decreased to avoid toxicity

(e) Toxicity is mainly bone marrow suppression

2. Fludarabine, hydroxyurea

(a) Both inhibit ribonucleotide reductase, a key enzyme in nucleotide synthesis in leukocytes

(b) Both are therefore chiefly used for leukemias

(c) Both cause bone marrow depression, although hydroxyurea causes mild bone marrow suppression that is dose-related and thus easily titratable, which makes **hydroxyurea an ideal chronic maintenance therapy to maintain normal cell counts in lymphoproliferative diseases** (e.g., chronic myeloid leukemia [CML], essential thrombocythemia, polycythemia vera)

(d) Hydroxyurea also induces the synthesis of high-affinity, fetal hemoglobin, and has shown benefit in sickle cell disease by reducing the frequency of crises

3. Cladribine

(a) Causes fragmentation of DNA strands

(b) Useful for hairy cell leukemia

(c) Causes bone marrow suppression

E. Pyrimidine antagonists

1. 5-fluorouracil (5-FU) & capecitabine (Xeloda)

(a) 5-FU is a prodrug converted intracellularly to an analog that prevents thymine synthesis by inhibiting thymidylate synthetase

- (b) Folinic acid (leucovorin) increases the binding of 5-FU to thymidylate synthetase, thereby potentiating the antitumor effect of 5-FU
- (c) Dose-limiting toxicities are mucositis/diarrhea and bone marrow suppression
- (d) It is chiefly used for adenocarcinomas, particularly of the colon, but also for rectal, gastric, and head and neck cancers
- (e) Capecitabine is an oral agent that is converted to 5-FU in vivo and can be used for oral, outpatient therapy of adenocarcinomas

2. Gemcitabine
   - (a) A prodrug converted in vivo to a nucleotide analog that is incorporated into DNA and causes chain termination
   - (b) Can cause severe bone marrow suppression, severe diarrhea, and mucositis
   - (c) A highly active drug used currently as salvage therapy for a variety of incurable GI adenocarcinomas, especially pancreatic cancer, and lung cancer

3. Cytarabine (ara-C)
   - (a) A prodrug converted in vivo to a nucleotide analog that inhibits DNA polymerase
   - (b) Causes severe bone marrow suppression, alopecia, mucositis, and peripheral neuropathy
   - (c) At high doses it is the 1st-line chemotherapy agent (equivalent to bone marrow transplant in many studies) for acute myelogenous leukemia (AML)

4. Azacytidine
   - (a) A nucleoside analogue of cytidine
   - (b) First treatment indicated specifically for myelodysplastic syndrome
   - (c) Works by inducing DNA hypomethylation and direct cidal effects

5. Bortezomib
   - (a) **First in class, inhibitor of the cellular proteosome—NOT a monoclonal antibody**
   - (b) Proteosome degrades ubiquinated proteins, and inhibition of the proteosome causes buildup of cellular toxins that lead to induction of apoptosis
   - (c) Works for refractory multiple myeloma

IV. Plant Derivatives (see Table 10.1)

A. Vinca alkaloids

1. Vincristine (Oncovin) and vinblastine are the chief drugs; vinorelbine (Navelbine) also in use

2. **They are of similar structure and identical mechanism: they poison the mitotic spindle by causing depolymerization of microtubules and thus arrest cell division in metaphase of mitosis**

3. Despite these similarities, they have different major toxicities and clinical efficacy

4. Vincristine

    (a) Used for lymphoma therapy as part of CHOP and MOPP, and is used for leukemias

    (b) **Major toxicity is peripheral neuropathy,** including neuropathic pain, weakness, and loss of reflexes

5. Vinblastine

    (a) Used for germ cell tumors and lymphoma as part of ABVD regimen

    (b) **Major toxicity is bone marrow suppression, and neurotoxicity is unusual**

6. Vinorelbine is primarily used as salvage therapy for breast cancer

B. Podophyllotoxin

1. VP-16 (etoposide) is the major drug in this class

2. Causes DNA strand rupture by inhibiting topoisomerase II

3. Major toxicities include bone marrow suppression, alopecia, nausea, vomiting

4. Used in small-cell lung cancer and for testicular cancer

C. Taxanes

1. Paclitaxel (Taxol) and docetaxel (Taxotere) are the major drugs in this class

2. **They act by promoting microtubule assembly and inhibiting microtubule disassembly, thereby inducing apoptosis**

3. Dose-limiting toxicity is bone marrow suppression, but can also cause peripheral neuropathy

4. Major uses are in breast, lung, and ovarian cancers

V. Endocrine Therapies (see Table 10.1)

A. Tamoxifen

1. An estrogen receptor agonist-antagonist that specifically antagonizes estrogen receptors found in breast tissue
2. Side effects include hot flashes, increased risk of thromboembolic disease/strokes, and a low incidence of endometrial cancer
3. Tamoxifen has revolutionized the therapy for breast cancer
   (a) **As primary prophylaxis, tamoxifen drastically lowers the risk of breast cancer developing in women at high risk**
   (b) **Tamoxifen drastically lowers the risk of breast cancer recurrence and is used as adjuvant therapy for 5 years**

B. Prednisone and dexamethasone

1. Primarily used for lymphomas and lymphocytic leukemias, directly induce lymphocyte cell death
2. Prednisone is used as part of MOPP and CHOP, dexamethasone as part of more intensive regimens
3. Major adverse effects are induction or exacerbation of diabetes, fluid retention, hypertension, immunosuppression, poor wound healing

C. Leuprolide

1. Synthetic analog of gonadotropin-releasing hormone (GnRH)
2. When given continuously, it feedback-suppresses the synthesis/release of sex hormones
3. Thus it is used for prostate cancer, which is androgen-dependent for growth
4. Toxicity is mild, mostly hot flashes

D. Flutamide

1. Antagonizes testosterone receptor
2. Used to treat metastatic prostate cancer
3. Causes gynecomastia

VI. Biological Response Modifiers

A. Vitamins

1. All-trans-retinoic acid (ATRA)
   (a) Binds to the mutated, fusion receptor for retinoic acid formed by the chromosome 15:17 translocation seen in AML, subtype M_3

(b) **ATRA causes a reactivation of the differentiation cascade in the blast cells, leading them to differentiate into more mature myeloid cells**

(c) This can induce remission in up to 90% of AML M$_3$ patients

(d) **Major toxicity is ATRA syndrom-respiratory distress from a combination of pneumonitis, pleural effusion, and pericardial effusion, treated with steriods**

B. Monoclonal antibodies

1. Rituximab (Rituxan)

(a) **An anti-CD20 monoclonal antibody**

(b) CD20 is a pan-B-cell marker, so rituximab has been used as adjunct therapy with CHOP for lymphomas, and data are now available indicating that responses are improved with the addition of rituximab

(c) It is also being investigated in a variety of collagen vascular diseases and autoimmune diseases thought to be mediated by autoantibody production

2. Trastuzumab (Herceptin)

(a) An antibody directed against the protein product of the *Her-2-neu* gene, which is **overexpressed in some breast cancers**

(b) Improves outcomes in breast cancers that do overexpress the gene

3. Gemtuzumab (Mylotarg)

(a) A monoclonal antibody directed against the CD33 surface protein, which is expressed on myeloid cells, and covalently linked to a toxic chemotherapeutic agent (calicheamicin)

(b) Used for AML; the monoclonal antibody targets the toxic agent to myeloid blast cells

4. Alemtuzumab: anti-CD52 monoclonal antibody for Chronic Lymphocytic Leukemia

5. Tositumomab

(a) Anti-CD20 monoclonal antibody, different from rituximab, linked to radioactive iodine

(b) Used for non-Hodgkin's lymphoma

6. Ibritumomab

(a) Anti-CD20 monoclonal antibody, different from rituximab and tositumomab, linked to radioactive indium or yttrium

(b) Used for non-Hodgkin's lymphoma

7. Bevacizumab
   (a) Anti-vascular endothelial growth factor (VEGF) monoclonal antibody
   (b) Blocks angiogenesis, for metastatic colon CA
8. Cetuximab: anti-epidermal growth factor (EGF) monoclonal antibody for metastatic colon CA

C. Cytokines
   1. Interleukin-2 is used in combination with surgery to treat renal cell carcinoma and melanoma, can cause capillary leak syndrome
   2. Interferon-α is used to treat hairy cell leukemia, chronic myelogenous leukemia, and Kaposi's sarcoma with encouraging rates of remission, but causes flulike illness and can cause severe depression
   3. Granulocyte-colony stimulating factor (G-CSF) and granulocyte-monocyte (GM-CSF) are used to support bone marrow in patients receiving myelotoxic chemotherapy

D. Enzyme inhibitors
   1. Imatinib mesylate (Gleevec)
      (a) A selective tyrosine kinase inhibitor
      (b) Specifically inhibits the constitutive tyrosine kinase created by the *bcr-abl* translocation seen in chronic myeloid leukemia (CML), thereby inhibiting the growth of the leukemic cell—it is FDA-approved for use in CML in blast crisis or accelerated phase, or as 2nd-line therapy in interferon-α failures
      (c) Also appears to have activity in some solid tumors

11. ANTIMICROBIALS

I. Principles

A. Antimicrobial agents are toxins that are more selective for microbial biochemistry than human biochemistry

B. The choice of appropriate antibiotic depends on several factors
1. Spectrum of coverage—know the general spectrum of microbes covered by each agent
2. Toxicity—in general, toxicities are class-specific; that is, toxicity depends on the class of antibiotic more than the individual agent, but some toxicities are agent-specific, and you should know these
3. Pharmacokinetics—some drugs penetrate certain tissues and body fluids better than others; some cannot be given orally and others cannot be given IV
4. Cidal versus static
   (a) Cidal antibiotics directly induce microbial cell death
   (b) Static antibiotics inhibit microbial growth but do not directly cause death
   (c) In patients with normal immune systems, static drugs are acceptable because the drugs slow the microbes enough for the immune system to catch up
   (d) **For immunocompromised patients cidal drugs are often preferred because theoretically static drugs may not clear the infection**
5. Synergy—some antibiotic combinations are known for synergy (e.g., β-lactam plus aminoglycoside), and these combinations should be favored when possible

C. The minimum inhibitory concentration (MIC)
1. The MIC is the concentration of antibiotic required to inhibit visible growth of the target bacteria in the test tube
2. For example, if the MIC of gentamicin for a certain *P. aeruginosa* strain is 0.5 µg/mL, growth of that strain in the test tube will occur if the gentamicin concentration is < 0.5 µg/mL, but not if the concentration is ≥ 0.5 µg/mL
3. By comparing the MIC in the test tube with the achievable levels of antibiotics in the body, general determinations of in vivo efficacy can be determined
4. For example, because peak gentamicin levels in the bloodstream are 5–10 µg/mL, a *P. aeruginosa* strain with a gentamicin MIC of 0.5 µg/mL would be considered "susceptible" to gentamicin,

and gentamicin could be used to treat a patient with a bloodstream infection caused by this strain

5. However, in the real world, just knowing the MIC value is not enough to predict efficacy in infected patients, because other factors complicate the outcome (e.g., if the bacteria is infecting a part of the body where the antibiotic does not penetrate well, blood levels of the antibiotic will not predict efficacy, and tissue levels must be known)

D. Antibiotics can be classified as concentration-dependent or time-dependent killers

1. Concentration-dependent killers
   (a) Efficacy depends on how high the peak serum concentration of the antibiotic is above the MIC and does not depend on how long the concentration remains above the MIC
   (b) When dosing concentration-dependent killers, the emphasis is placed on less frequent administration of higher drug amounts to maximize the peak serum level
   (c) For example, it is ideal to dose aminoglycosides at high doses only once per day even though the drugs have short half-lives, as this maximizes the peak level
   (d) Concentration-dependent killers have a "postantibiotic effect," in which the bacteria continue to die even after the level of the antibiotic falls below the bacteria's MIC
   (e) Concentration-dependent killers include aminoglycosides, fluoroquinolones, daptomycin, and telithromycin

2. Time-dependent killers
   (a) Efficacy depends on how long the concentration of the antibiotic remains above the bacteria's MIC and is unrelated to how high above the MIC the antibiotic concentration is
   (b) When dosing time-dependent killers, emphasis is placed on more frequent dosing of lower drug amounts, to maximize the time above the MIC
   (c) Time-dependent killers include all β lactam antibiotics (e.g. penicillins, cephalosporins, monobactams, carbapenems) and vancomycin

3. Cmax/MIC, Time Above MIC, AUC/MIC
   (a) It is increasingly popular to rationally dose antibiotics based on knowledge of their pharmacodynamics
   (b) Cmax/MIC
       (1) For pure concentration-dependent killers, activity can be predicted by knowing the peak serum level (Cmax) divided by the bacteria's MIC (Cmax/MIC)

(2) The desired Cmax/MIC ratio differs for different antibiotics and different bacteria

(3) For example, the desired aminoglycoside Cmax/MIC ratio is ≥10, and in fact activity continues to improve as the Cmax/MIC ratio increases from 10 to 30 (if the MIC is 0.5 μg/mL, desired peak serum level is ≥5 μg/mL, and activity will continue to improve up to a peak serum level of 15 μg/mL)

(c) Time Above MIC

(1) For pure time-dependent killers, activity can be predicted by knowing what fraction of the dosing interval the antibiotic concentration remains above the MIC (the Time Above MIC)

(2) For β lactams, the desired Time Above MIC is >50% of the dosing interval, but activity may continue to improve if the Time Above MIC equals the entire dosing interval

(3) For example, if the MIC of the target bacteria is 1 μg/mL and the β lactam antibiotic is dosed every 8 hours, you want the serum level of the β lactam to remain above 1 μg/mL for at least 4 hours, and preferably for the entire 8-hour period

(d) AUC/MIC

(1) It is intuitive that the single best predictor of most antibiotics should be the total exposure of the bacteria to the antibiotic, which cannot be simply described by Cmax/MIC or Time Above MIC

(2) The AUC/MIC is an integrated calculation of the "area under the curve" of serum levels, or the total amount of drug in the bloodstream over the dosing interval, divided by the MIC

(3) Because the AUC/MIC ratio takes into consideration BOTH concentration and time-dependent activity, the AUC/MIC is the single-best predictor of in vivo activity of most antibiotics

II. Antiseptics

A. Ethanol

1. Rapidly acting and cidal, but not especially effective

2. Most useful at removing layers of dead skin and dander to allow other antimicrobials to work better

B. Chlorhexidine
1. Rapidly acting, cidal, broad spectrum of activity, highly effective antimicrobial
2. Causes minimal skin irritation

C. Iodine
1. Typically delivered in complex with a carrier molecule (e.g., povidone)
2. Highly effective, cidal when solution dries on skin
3. Can cause marked irritation to skin if left on for prolonged periods

III. Bacterial Cell Wall Inhibitors

A. Penicillins (see Table 11.1 for individual agents)
1. Mechanism: **inhibit bacterial cell wall synthesis** by blocking the **transpeptidase**-dependent cross-linkage of peptidoglycan
2. Resistance: several mechanisms described
   (a) β-**lactamase production:** many bacteria express β-lactamase, an enzyme that cleaves open the four-membered β-lactam ring in penicillins, inactivating them—**this can be overcome by adding a β-lactamase inhibitor to the penicillin**, which protects the penicillin from the bacterial β-lactamase
   (b) Altered penicillin binding proteins (PBPs): some bacteria have mutated penicillin binding targets (the transpeptidases); this is the mechanism for methicillin-resistant *Staphylococcus aureus* (MRSA)
3. Toxicities: hypersensitivity reactions (including anaphylaxis) common, can also see leukopenia and can induce autoimmune hemolytic anemia
4. Cidal/static: cidal for actively dividing bacteria
5. Coverage:
   (a) Simple penicillin: coverage limited to *Strep* agents and oral anaerobes
   (b) Aminopenicillins: improved gram-positive and anaerobic coverage, adds some community-acquired gram-negative rod (GNR) coverage
   (c) β-lactamase inhibitors: when added to aminopenicillins these dramatically enhance coverage of gram positives (e.g., *Staphylococcus*), community GNR, and anaerobes

Table 11.1 Penicillins

Drug	Subclass	Characteristics
penicillin	Penicillin	• Covers *Streptococcus*, oral anaerobes, syphilis • Good for strep throat, oral/dental infections
ampicillin	Aminopenicillin	• Also covers *Enterococcus*, *Listeria*, some GNR • Only given intravenously
amoxicillin	Aminopenicillin	• As per ampicillin, but good oral absorption
ampicillin + sulbactam	Aminopenicillin + β-lactamase inhibitor	• Sulbactam inhibits bacterial β-lactamase • Adds *Staph*, community GNR, & anaerobic coverage
amoxicillin + clavulanate	Aminopenicillin + β-lactamase inhibitor	• Clavulanate inhibits bacterial β-lactamase • Per ampicillin + sulbactam, but oral instead of parenteral
methicillin	Penicillinase-resistant penicillin	• Specifically designed to cover *Staph* • Too toxic for general use, causing interstitial nephritis • Used in the lab to define MRSA, which has altered penicillin-binding proteins and thus cannot be treated with any β-lactam
oxacillin nafcillin	Penicillinase-resistant penicillin	• Derivatives of methicillin that are less toxic • 1st-line therapy for methicillin-susceptible *S. aureus* (MSSA)
dicloxacillin	Penicillinase-resistant penicillin	• Oral version of oxacillin
piperacillin	Ureidopenicillin	• Covers *Strep* and GNR, including *Pseudomonas*/nosocomial GNR
ticarcillin	Carboxypenicillin	• Similar to piperacillin
piperacillin + tazobactam	Ureidopenicillin + β-lactamase inhibitor	• Adds MSSA and anaerobic bacteria, broader GNR
ticarcillin + clavulanate	Carboxypenicillin + β-lactamase inhibitor	• Similar to piperacillin + tazobactam

(d) Penicillinase-resistant penicillins: best methicillin susceptible *S. aureus* (MSSA) coverage of all penicillins, but does not cover methicillin resistant *S. aureus* (MRSA)

(e) Ureidopenicillins: broad spectrum coverage, including nosocomial GNR

B. Cephalosporins (see Table 11.2 for individual agents)

1. <u>Mechanism</u>: like penicillins, **inhibit bacterial cell wall synthesis** by blocking the transpeptidase-dependent cross-linkage of peptidoglycan

Table 11.2 Cephalosporins

Drug	Generation	Characteristics
cefazolin	1st	• Very good MSSA & *Strep* coverage, OK for community GNR • Good agent for skin infections (but no MRSA coverage), also for community UTIs • Only administered IV
cephalexin	1st	• An oral agent similar to cefazolin
cefuroxime	2nd	• Better *Strep* but worse MSSA, better for community GNR • One of the few agents that can be both oral and IV
cefamandole	2nd	• Contains a methylthiotetrazole (MTT) side chain • MTT interferes with vitamin K–dependent γ-carboxylation → prolonged PT & also causes disulfiram-like reaction to EtOH • It is rarely used clinically, but a classic USMLE topic
cefotetan	2nd	• Loses MSSA coverage, good community GNR, but the key is outstanding anaerobic coverage • Also has an MTT moiety → ↑ PT and disulfiram-like effects
cefoxitin	2nd	• Similar to cefotetan but lacks the MTT moiety
ceftriaxone	3rd	• Best *Strep* coverage of all cephalosporins, loses most of MSSA coverage, excellent community GNR but no nosocomial GNR coverage

Table 11.2 (Continued)

Drug	Generation	Characteristics
		• Key to this drug is once a day dosing (24 hr effect)—1st line for meningitis, also for pneumonia, urinary infections
cefotaxime	3rd	• Similar to ceftriaxone but doses 3×/day (8 hr effect)
ceftizoxime	3rd	• Similar to cefotaxime but has expanded anaerobic coverage
ceftazidime	3rd	• Loses all gram-positive coverage, but has excellent *Pseudomonas* coverage, excellent nosocomial GNR
cefixime	3rd	• An oral agent, good for MSSA, *Strep*, and community GNR
cefepime	4th	• Remarkably broad spectrum, excellent MSSA, *Strep*, community and nosocomial GNR

2. <u>Resistance</u>: two major mechanisms
   (a) β-lactamase production: some β-lactamase enzymes destroy cephalosporins, which also contain the four-membered β-lactam ring
   (b) Altered penicillin binding proteins
3. <u>Toxicities</u>: hypersensitivity reactions less common than with penicillins and **only 15% cross-reactivity between penicillin allergy and cephalosporin allergy**; cephalosporins also can cause biliary sludging
4. <u>Cidal/static</u>: cidal for actively dividing bacteria
5. <u>Coverage</u>:
   (a) <u>1st generation</u>: very good MSSA and *Strep* coverage, OK community GNR
   (b) <u>2nd generation</u>: better *Strep* coverage but worse *Staph* coverage, better community GNR, better anaerobic coverage
   (c) <u>3rd generation</u>: gram-positive coverage varies by drug, but all have improved GNR coverage, and some cover nosocomial GNR, **all penetrate CNS better than 1st or 2nd generation and therefore are preferred for meningitis**

ANTIMICROBIALS

C. Carbapenems (see Table 11.3 for individual agents)

1. <u>Mechanism</u>: like penicillins, **inhibit bacterial cell wall synthesis by blocking the transpeptidase-dependent cross-linkage of peptidoglycan**

2. <u>Resistance</u>: β-lactamases don't work well against carbapenems so this is not a mechanism of resistance; however, altered penicillin binding proteins still a problem

3. <u>Toxicities</u>: seizures

4. <u>Cidal/static</u>: cidal for actively dividing bacteria

5. <u>Coverage</u>: **probably the broadest-spectrum coverage available in any single agents**

D. Monobactams (see Table 11.3 for individual agents)

1. <u>Mechanism</u>: like penicillins, **inhibit bacterial cell wall synthesis** by blocking the transpeptidase-dependent cross-linkage of peptidoglycan

2. <u>Resistance</u>: β-lactamases don't work well against monobactams, so this is not a mechanism of resistance; however, altered penicillin binding proteins still a problem

3. <u>Toxicities</u>: minimal, no cross-reactivity to penicillins

4. <u>Cidal/static</u>: cidal for actively dividing bacteria

5. <u>Coverage</u>: excellent GNR coverage

E. Glycopeptide and lipopeptide (see Table 11.3 for individual agents)

1. <u>Mechanism</u>:

   (a) Glycopeptides inhibit cell wall synthesis, **vancomycin acts by binding to D-alanine-D-alanine subunits and preventing their insertion into the cell wall**

   (b) The lipopeptide daptomycin punches holes in the cell membrane, creating pores that cause leakage of intracellular ions leading to depolarizing the cellular membrane and inhibition of macromolecular synthesis

2. <u>Resistance</u>: all gram negatives are intrinsically resistant to all of these agents, gram-positive resistance is unusual to date, although vancomycin-resistant *Enterococcus* (VRE) is now quite common

3. <u>Toxicities</u>:

   (a) Vancomycin classic toxicity is the **"red man syndrome"** = **histamine reaction → skin turns red**

   (b) Daptomycin is well tolerated; if dosed inappropriately (twice daily) myositis is common, but myositis is rare with once daily dosing

Table 11.3 Carbapenems, Monobactams, & Glycopeptides

Drug	Class	Characteristics
imipenem	Carbapenem	• Hits everything except intracellular bacteria • Can cause seizures • Inactivated by dihydropeptidase enzyme in renal tubular cells, so administered with another agent, cilastatin, which prevents degradation in renal cells, thereby prolonging imipenem effects
meropenem	Carbapenem	• Similar spectrum to imipenem, less prone to induce seizures
ertapenem	Carbapenem	• Less broad spectrum than imipenem and meropenem • Covers MSSA, *Strep*, community GNR, and anaerobes, but does not cover *Pseudomonas* or some other nosocomial GNR
aztreonam	Monobactam	• No gram-positive coverage, no anaerobic coverage, excellent GNR coverage including nosocomials
vancomycin	Glycopeptide	• Covers almost all gram-positive cocci, including MRSA, but not vancomycin-resistant *Enterococcus* (VRE)
bacitracin	Glycopeptide	• Topical agent
dalbavancin	Glycopeptide	• Similar spectrum to vancomycin but also covers VRE • Incredibly long half-life allows **dosing once per week** • Not yet FDA approved (anticipated in 2005–2006)
daptomycin	Lipopeptide	• First in class agent, the most rapidly cidal agent known for gram positives • Covers almost all gram positives, including MRSA and VRE • Watch for myositis (rarely seen with daily dosing but common with twice daily dosing)

ANTIMICROBIALS

4. Cidal/static: vancomycin is static, daptomycin is cidal
5. Coverage: cover almost all gram positives, with daptomycin and dalbavancin covering VRE also, but none of these drugs cover gram negatives

IV. Folate Antagonists (see Table 11.4 for summary)

A. Trimethoprim
   1. Mechanism: **trimethoprim blocks dihydrofolate reductase,** inhibiting generation of folate
   2. Resistance: mutations in the folate synthetic pathway and in the enzyme targets
   3. Toxicities: minimal toxicities
   4. Cidal/static: static
   5. Coverage: covers many gram-positive cocci (GPC) and some GNR

B. Sulfonamides
   1. Mechanism: **act as structural analogs for para-aminobenzoic acid (PABA), a folate precursor, inhibiting folate synthesis**
   2. Resistance: mutations in the folate synthetic pathway and in the enzyme targets
   3. Toxicities: all sulfa drugs are prone to inducing allergic reactions, ranging from rash to anaphylaxis
   4. Cidal/static: static
   5. Coverage: covers many GPC and some GNR, as well as atypical organisms like *Nocardia*

C. Trimethoprim/sulfamethoxazole (Bactrim)
   1. Mechanism: **synergistic block of the folate synthetic pathway**
   2. Resistance: mutations in the folate synthetic pathway and in the enzyme targets

Table 11.4 Folate Antagonists

Drug	Characteristics
trimethoprim	• Broad spectrum activity, but static; nontoxic
sulfonamides	• Broad spectrum activity, but static, allergic reactions common
trimethoprim-sulfamethoxazole	• Synergistic inhibition of folate synthesis → cidal, allergic reactions common

3. <u>Toxicities</u>: similar to sulfonamides, allergic reactions common
4. <u>Cidal/static</u>: cidal (ain't synergy grand!)
5. <u>Coverage</u>: covers GPC, GNR, and atypicals well, and its concentration in the kidney, urine, and prostate make it ideal for uncomplicated UTIs, kidney infections, and GU infections

V. Protein Synthesis Inhibitors (see Table 11.5 for individual agents)

A. Aminoglycosides
  1. <u>Mechanism</u>: **binds to 30S subunit of bacterial ribosome, blocking protein synthesis initiation and causing misreading of the mRNA code**
  2. <u>Resistance</u>: several major mechanisms described
     (a) Altered uptake of the drug
     (b) Bacterial enzymes add acetyl groups to aminoglycosides, modifying the drugs' structures, thereby inactivating them
     (c) Mutations in bacterial ribosomes, blocking the drugs' ability to bind to their targets
     (d) Anaerobes are intrinsically resistant, as aminoglycosides require an oxidative environment to be transported into the cell
  3. <u>Toxicities</u>:
     (a) **Renal tubular damage and ototoxicity are the most prominent toxicities**
     (b) Toxicity is related to the amount of time the serum levels exceed a certain concentration
     (c) Conversely, efficacy is proportional to the peak serum concentration, irrespective of how long the drug levels are high
     (d) **This is because of the postantibiotic effect, in which aminoglycosides continue killing bacteria for hours after the drug falls below its "therapeutic" concentration**
     (e) Maximizing efficacy requires a high peak serum level, and minimizing toxicity requires spending most of the dosing interval with serum concentration low
     (f) **Therefore, administration of aminoglycosides is almost always once a day now, versus three times a day in the past, achieving a high peak dose and allowing the levels to fall below toxic levels for the remainder of the day**

ANTIMICROBIALS

Table 11.5 Protein Synthesis Inhibitors

Drug	Class	Characteristics
streptomycin	Aminoglycoside	• Sometimes used to treat *Mycobacteria* • Seldom used due to more resistance than to other agents
gentamicin	Aminoglycoside	• Excellent for GNR, predominant toxicity is renal failure
amikacin	Aminoglycoside	• Frequently active even against organisms resistant to other aminoglycosides • Commonly causes both ototoxicity and nephrotoxicity
tobramycin	Aminoglycoside	• Often used in inhaled form for pts with cystic fibrosis who develop *Pseudomonas* infections • Can cause both renal and ototoxicity
neomycin	Aminoglycoside	• Too toxic for parenteral use but poorly orally absorbed • Given orally to sterilize the bowel prior to bowel surgery, and to reduce the concentration of colonic flora, thereby reducing the synthesis of ammonium compounds in the gut in pts with hepatic encephalopathy
tetracycline	Tetracycline	• Used principally for acne; oral absorption is variable
doxycycline	Tetracycline	• Excellent oral absorption, most commonly used tetracycline
demeclocycline	Tetracycline	• Causes nephrogenic diabetes insipidus, which can be useful for patients with hyponatremia 2° to SIADH
tigecycline	Glycylcycline (tetracycline derivative)	• Much broader than all other tetracyclines • Addition of *N-t*-butyl-glycylamido group to minocycline nucleus prevents efflux of drug from GNR • Covers the dreaded *Acinetobacter*, MRSA, VRE, nosocomial GNR, but not *Pseudomonas*
chloramphenicol	Chloramphenicol	• Rarely used in developed world, 2° idiosyncratic toxicity

Table 11.5 (Continued)

Drug	Class	Characteristics
		• Still useful in underdeveloped countries due to broad spectrum of activity, excellent CNS penetration, & low cost
erythromycin	Macrolide	• Used for pneumonia because it covers *Strep* and atypicals such as *Mycoplasma* and *Legionella* • Drug of choice to treat penicillin-sensitive infections in penicillin-allergic patients
clarithromycin	Macrolide	• Much better tolerated, coverage of *Strep* and atypicals similar to erythromycin • 1st line to cover *Helicobacter pylori* and *Mycobacterium avium intracellulare* • Also useful for pneumonia treatment
azithromycin	Macrolide	• Per clarithromycin, but is 1st line to prophylax AIDS pts for *Mycobacterium avium intracellulare* • Once a day dosing, with half-life > 24 hrs • Also useful for pneumonia treatment
telithromycin	Ketolide (macrolide derivative)	• Covers most gram-positive organisms including all *Strep* (including drug-resistant *S. pneumonia*), some MRSA, and excellent atypical coverage • Used for community acquired pneumonia
clindamycin	Lincosamide	• 1st line for anaerobic coverage above the diaphragm • 2nd line for skin infections, good *Staph/Strep* coverage
quinupristin/ dalfopristin	Streptogramin	• Broad spectrum gram-positive coverage, including VRE and MRSA, but no gram-negative coverage
linezolid	Oxazolidinone	• Covers all GPC, including VRE & MRSA

4. Cidal/static: cidal
5. Coverage: first-line agents for gram negatives, excellent nosocomial GNR coverage, **synergize with cell-wall inhibitors to kill GPC**, do not cover anaerobes at all

B. Tetracyclines/glycylcycline
   1. Mechanism: **bind to 30S subunit of bacterial ribosome, blocking the acceptor site for the incoming aminoacyl-tRNA, thereby inhibiting protein synthesis**
   2. Resistance: due to decreased uptake or actual efflux of the drug from the bacteria mediated by a pump protein
   3. Toxicities: discoloration of teeth in children, photosensitize skin → sunburns
   4. Cidal/static: static
   5. Coverage: fairly broad spectrum, covering GPC and some GNR, but most useful for intracellular, atypical bacteria—the glycylcycline tigecycline has markedly expanded coverage due to prevention of drug efflux by the N-t-butyl substitution on the minocycline nucleus, adding MRSA, VRE, and *Acinetobacter* coverage
   6. Absorption: **tetracycline absorption in the gut is inhibited by divalent or trivalent cations, including Ca^{2+}, Mg^{2+}, and Al^{3+}, commonly found in antacids**

C. Chloramphenicol
   1. Mechanism: **binds to the 50S subunit of bacterial ribosome, blocking the action of peptidyltransferase, which inhibits formation of the peptide bond**
   2. Resistance: most common mechanism is acetylation of the drug, which inactivates it; can also be due to decreased drug uptake
   3. Toxicities:
      (a) Dose-dependent aplastic anemia, reversible with cessation of the drug
      (b) **Idiosyncratic aplastic anemia, not reversible after drug cessation** and not related to total dose of drug given; **interestingly it has mostly been reported after oral administration of the drug**, with very few cases worldwide after intravenous administration
      (c) **Gray-baby syndrome is due to uncoupling of oxidative phosphorylation** in the myocardium in infants, causing cyanosis and shock

4. Cidal/static: static
5. Coverage: very broad spectrum activity, including gram positives, many community GNRs, atypical/intracellular organisms, and many anaerobes, but not considered 1st line for infections in the developed world

D. Macrolides/ketolide

1. Mechanism: **binds to 50S subunit of bacterial ribosome and blocks translocation of amino acids, interfering with protein synthesis**

2. Resistance: due to decreased cell uptake, enzymatic inactivation of the drugs, or mutations affecting the drugs' binding site on the ribosome

3. Toxicities: GI upset with nausea, vomiting, and diarrhea is very common with erythromycin, **drug interactions with agents metabolized by cytochrome P450 (such as antihistamines) causes QT prolongation which can lead to torsade de pointes**

4. Cidal/static: macrolides static, the ketolide telithromycin is cidal

5. Coverage:
   (a) 1st generation: covers *Strep* and atypicals but has no gram-negative coverage
   (b) 2nd generation: much better tolerated (fewer GI adverse effects), have excellent *Strep* and atypical coverage, but still minimal gram-negative coverage—the ketolide telithromycin binds much more tightly to the target site than macrolides, and therefore covers even macrolide resistant *S. pneumonia* and some MRSA

E. Lincosamide

1. Mechanism: **binds to 50S subunit of bacterial ribosome and blocks formation of peptide bond**

2. Resistance: due to mutations altering the drug's binding site on the bacterial ribosomes

3. Toxicities: **major risk is the triggering of *Clostridium difficile*** infection by wiping out the enteric flora, occurring in up to 10% of patients

4. Cidal/static: cidal for gram-positive cocci, static for anaerobes

5. Coverage: **1st line for anaerobic infections in the lung or oropharynx**, good 2nd-line agent for bowel anaerobes (behind metronidazole), also good activity against GPC (e.g., for skin infections)

ANTIMICROBIALS

F. Streptogramins
  1. Mechanism: **bind to the 50S subunit of bacterial ribosomes,** inhibiting protein synthesis
  2. Resistance: gram negatives and *Enterococcus faecalis* intrinsically resistant
  3. Toxicities: severe thrombophlebitis, requires central venous access
  4. Cidal/static: static
  5. Coverage: **covers most gram positives, including vancomycin-resistant** *Enterococcus* **(VRE)** (but not *E. faecalis*, fortunately most VRE is *E. faecium*), **and MRSA**

G. Oxazolidinone
  1. Mechanism: **binds to the 50S subunit of bacterial ribosomes,** inhibiting protein synthesis by a unique mechanism: it **prevents union of the 50S and 30S subunits into the 70S preinitiation complex,** thereby stopping protein synthesis before it ever begins
  2. Resistance: case reports of rare *Enterococcus* resistance
  3. Toxicities: anemia and thrombocytopenia
  4. Cidal/static: static
  5. Coverage: **covers essentially all GPC**

VI. Nucleic Acid Inhibitors (see Table 11.6 for individual agents)

A. Fluoroquinolones
  1. Mechanism: **blocks activity of DNA gyrase,** which unwinds bacterial DNA during genomic replication
  2. Resistance: due to mutations in DNA gyrase, making it resistant to the drugs' activity
  3. Toxicities: may cause bone or joint disease in children (only convincingly demonstrated in experimental animals), including tendon rupture
  4. Cidal/static: cidal
  5. Coverage: excellent gram-negative coverage, including nosocomial GNR, excellent coverage for atypical, intracellular infections (especially *Legionella*), & newer agents have gram-positive coverage as well

Table 11.6 Nucleic Acid Inhibitors

Drug	Class	Characteristics
ciprofloxacin	Fluoroquinolone	• Although it's the oldest fluoro-quinolone, it still has the best GNR coverage of all the drugs in the class • Chief use is in urine, prostate, bone, or blood infections caused by GNR
ofloxacin	Fluoroquinolone	• Good GNR and some GPC coverage • Uses similar to ciprofloxacin
levofloxacin	Fluoroquinolone	• Excellent *Strep* coverage, some *Staph* coverage, good GNR • Levofloxacin is the L-enantiomer of ofloxacin • Uses similar to ciprofloxacin, but can also be used for pneumonia or other *severe Strep. pneumonia* infections
moxifloxacin	Fluoroquinolone	• Newer generation agent, has expanded *Staph* and *Strep* coverage • Uses similar to ciprofloxacin, but can also be used for pneumonia or other severe *S. pneumoniae* infections
gatifloxacin	Fluoroquinolone	• As per moxifloxacin
gemifloxacin	Fluoroquinolone	• Similar to gatifloxacin
rifampin	Rifamycin	• Very broad spectrum activity but never used as monotherapy because of risk of resistance • Added to deep tissue infections because of its excellent tissue penetration, also used as part of TB therapy because of high intracellular concentrations
rifabutin	Rifamycin	• Similar to rifampin but less likely to interact with other medications, especially HIV antiviral agents
rifapentine	Rifamycin	• Similar to rifampin but long half-life allows once or twice weekly dosing

ANTIMICROBIALS

B. Rifamycins

1. Mechanism: **inhibit RNA polymerase**
2. Resistance: **resistance very commonly develops during monotherapy**, requiring that rifamycins always be given in combination with a 2nd agent; mechanism is mutation of bacterial RNA polymerase
3. Toxicities: **turns body secretions orange/red;** drug-induced hepatitis common
4. Cidal/static: cidal
5. Coverage: broad spectrum activity when combined with a second agent, **1st line as part of combination chemotherapy for TB**, useful as combination therapy for endocarditis or osteomyelitis because of **excellent tissue penetration**, used for close-contact prophylaxis in meningitis because of good salivary penetration

VII. Miscellaneous Agents (see Table 11.7 for individual agents)

A. Metronidazole

1. Mechanism: exact target unclear, but it **poisons anaerobic metabolism** and acts as an electron sink, depriving organisms of necessary reducing equivalents
2. Resistance: unusual, may be due to slow drug uptake
3. Toxicities: **has a disulfiram-like effect with alcohol, can cause a metallic aftertaste**
4. Cidal/static: cidal
5. Coverage: only drug in the class, **by far the most effective agent for all bowel anaerobes**, should be used for all biliary, hepatic, and bowel infections and all abscesses in the body

Table 11.7 Miscellaneous Agents

Drug	Characteristics
metronidazole	• 1st line for anaerobic infections, also covers protozoa like *Entamoeba*
isoniazid	• 1st line for TB therapy
ethambutol	• Used as part of four-drug therapy for TB
pyrazinamide	• Used as part of four-drug therapy for TB
dapsone	• 1st-line therapy for leprosy, 2nd line for *Pneumocystis carinii*

B. Isoniazid
   1. Mechanism: somehow **inhibits mycolic acid synthesis**
   2. Resistance: develops spontaneously in bacterial chromosomes at a certain set rate, so resistance develops during monotherapy if the organism burden in the patient is high enough to make it statistically possible
   3. Toxicities: **risk of fulminant hepatic toxicity, also commonly depletes vitamin B$_6$**
   4. Cidal/static: cidal
   5. Coverage: the only drug in the class, extremely effective for TB, also effective against other mycobacteria

C. Ethambutol
   1. Mechanism: unknown
   2. Resistance: unusual during combination drug therapy, but common during single-agent therapy, so single-agent therapy is never used
   3. Toxicities: **optic nerve and retinal toxicity** possible after long courses of therapy, and visual acuity should be regularly checked
   4. Cidal/static: cidal
   5. Coverage: the only drug in the class, used as part of four-drug therapy for TB (isoniazid, rifampin, ethambutol, pyrazinamide = RIPE drugs)

D. Pyrazinamide
   1. Mechanism: unclear
   2. Resistance: unusual during combination drug therapy
   3. Toxicities: hepatoxicity can develop
   4. Cidal/static: cidal
   5. Coverage: the only drug in the class, used as part of four-drug therapy for TB (RIPE drugs)

E. Dapsone
   1. Mechanism: unclear
   2. Resistance: will emerge during monotherapy for patients with large organism burden
   3. Toxicities: **hemolysis can occur, particularly in those with G6PDH deficiency;** methemoglobinemia and GI upset can also occur
   4. Cidal/static: cidal
   5. Coverage: the only drug in the class, used as 1st-line agent for leprosy, and 2nd-line agent for *Pneumocystis carinii*

Table 11.8 Summary of Antibacterial Antibiotic Classes

Class (Example)	Target	Process Inhibited	Toxicity	Key Coverage
penicillin (PCN)	transpeptidase	Cell wall synthesis	Allergic	*Strep*, oral anaerobes
aminopenicillin (ampicillin)	transpeptidase	Cell wall synthesis	Allergic	*Strep*, oral anaerobes, *Enterococcus, Listeria*
β-lactamase inhibitor + amp (amp/sulbactam)	transpeptidase	Cell wall synthesis	Allergic	GPC, GNR, anaerobes but not nosocomials
penicillinase-resistant PCN (oxacillin)	transpeptidase	Cell wall synthesis	Allergic	MSSA, some *Strep*
ureidopenicillin (piperacillin)	transpeptidase	Cell wall synthesis	Allergic	GPC, GNR, anaerobes, & nosocomials
1° cephalosporin (cefazolin)	transpeptidase	Cell wall synthesis	Allergic	MSSA/*Strep*, some GNR
2° cephalosporin (cefuroxime)	transpeptidase	Cell wall synthesis	Allergic	Better *Strep*, better GNR, worse MSSA
3° cephalosporin (ceftriaxone/ ceftazidime)	transpeptidase	Cell wall synthesis	Allergic	*Strep* & GNR, nosocomial (ceftazidime)
carbapenem (imipenem)	transpeptidase	Cell wall synthesis	Seizure	Broad coverage including nosocomials
monobactam (aztreonam)	transpeptidase	Cell wall synthesis	Minimal	GNR including nosocomials
glycopeptides (vancomycin)	D-alanine-D-alanine	Cell wall synthesis	Allergic	All GPC
lipopeptide (daptomycin)	bacterial membrane	Punch holes in membrane	Myositis (rare if dosed properly)	All GPC
aminoglycoside (gentamicin)	30S ribosome	Protein synthesis	Renal and ototoxic	GNR including nosocomials

Table 11.8 (Continued)

Class (Example)	Target	Process Inhibited	Toxicity	Key Coverage
tetracyclines (doxycycline)	30S ribosome	Protein synthesis	Bone/ teeth coloration	Atypicals
glycylcycline (tigecycline)	30S ribosome	Protein synthesis	Bone/ teeth coloration	MRSA, VRE, GNR, atypicals
chloramphenicol	50S ribosome	Protein synthesis	Bone marrow	Broad but not nosocomials
macrolide (erythromycin)	50S ribosome	Protein synthesis	GI upset	*Strep* and atypicals
ketolide (telithromycin)	50S ribosome	Protein synthesis	GI upset	*Strep* and atypicals
lincosamide (clindamycin)	50S ribosome	Protein synthesis	*C. difficile*	GPC, excellent for anaerobes
streptogramin (quinupristin/ dalfopristin)	50S ribosome	Protein synthesis	Thrombo- phlebitis	VRE & MRSA
oxazolidinone (linezolid)	50S ribosome	Protein synthesis	Anemia	All GPC
fluoroquinolones (ciprofloxacin)	DNA gyrase	DNA replication	Bone/joint damage	*Strep*, GNR, nosocomials, atypicals
trimethoprim-sulfamethoxazole	PABA/ dihydrofolate reductase	Folate synthesis	Allergic	GPC, GNR, protozoa
metronidazole	Unclear	Anaerobic metabolism	Minimal	1st line for anaerobes
rifamycins (rifampin)	RNA polymerase	RNA transcription	Red urine & tears	GPC, GNR, atypicals
isoniazid	Unclear	Mycolic acid synthesis	Hepatic, deplete B_6	*Mycobacteria*
ethambutol	Unclear	Unclear	Retinal	TB
pyrazinamide	Unclear	Unclear	Hepatic	TB
dapsone	Unclear	Unclear	Hemolysis	Leprosy

VIII. Antifungal Drugs (see Table 11.9 for individual agents)

Table 11.9 Antifungal Agents

Drug	Class	Characteristics
amphotericin B	Polyene	• 1st line for all severe fungal infections • Resistance is distinctly unusual, covers yeast and molds • Causes renal failure, type I renal tubular acidosis, potassium and magnesium wasting from kidney
liposomal amphotericin B & amphotericin B lipid complex	Polyene	• Similar activity to amphotericin B deoxycholate but less infusional and nephrotoxicity • Due to cost, reserve for use in patients with renal dysfunction
nystatin	Polyene	• Too toxic for parenteral use, poorly absorbed orally • Useful for thrush of oropharynx or esophagus
fluconazole	Azole	• 1st line for yeast infections, particularly *Candida* infections in a nonneutropenic host, *Cryptococcus*, and *Coccidioides* • Far superior safety profile vs. amphotericin, but it is not cidal and does not cover molds, so use cautiously in neutropenic patients
itraconazole	Azole	• Oral absorption is far more variable than fluconazole • Does cover some molds, especially *Aspergillus*
miconazole	Azole	• Used for topical fungal infections (e.g., athlete's foot)
clotrimazole	Azole	• Used for topical fungal infections (e.g., vaginal infections)
voriconazole	Azole	• Broad spectrum activity, much expanded from fluconazole, rivals amphotericin • In a head-to-head clinical trial, was superior to amphotericin for *Aspergillus* infections

Table 11.9 (Continued)

Drug	Class	Characteristics
		• Covers yeast and molds, except *Mucor* • Transient visual changes occur but resolve with continued therapy
5-flucytosine	Nucleoside analog	• Resistance develops with monotherapy; always used in combination with amphotericin
terbinafine	Allylamine	• Only used for onychomycosis (toenail infections) • Can cause hepatotoxicity
griseofulvin	Griseofulvin	• Only used for onychomycosis (toenail infections) • Can cause hepatotoxicity
caspofungin	Echinocandin	• Excellent *Candida* coverage, and covers *Aspergillus* • Virtually no side effects
micafungin	Echinocandin	• Coverage and side effects similar to caspofungin, but less clinical data available

A. Polyenes

   1. <u>Mechanism</u>: **bind to ergosterol in the fungal cell membrane,** punching holes in the membrane
   2. <u>Resistance</u>: unusual
   3. <u>Toxicities</u>: toxic parenteral agents, poorly tolerated by patients due to **severe rigors and malaise, also cause dose-dependent renal insufficiency and renal tubular acidosis with potassium and magnesium wasting**
   4. <u>Cidal/static</u>: cidal
   5. <u>Coverage</u>: **broadest spectrum antifungal agents available,** cover both yeasts and molds, 1st line for serious infections

B. Azoles

   1. <u>Mechanism</u>: **inhibit ergosterol synthesis by disrupting the cytochrome p450 pathway**
   2. <u>Resistance</u>: some species are intrinsically resistant due to altered p450 enzymes (e.g., *Candida krusei*), resistance is an increasingly common problem

3. <u>Toxicities</u>: GI intolerance, cholestasis, hepatitis are the most common
4. <u>Cidal/static</u>: static
5. <u>Coverage</u>: **azoles all cover yeast very well, but are static so must be used cautiously in neutropenic patients**—some members of the class cover molds as well

C. 5-flucytosine (5FC)

1. <u>Mechanism</u>: **inhibits DNA synthesis in fungal cells,** less so in human cells
2. <u>Resistance</u>: **is expected to develop if used as monotherapy, so it's always combined with a 2nd agent, typically amphotericin**
3. <u>Toxicities</u>: bone marrow suppression
4. <u>Cidal/static</u>: cidal
5. <u>Coverage</u>: 1st line for *Cryptococcus* meningitis in combination with amphotericin

D. Terbinafine

1. <u>Mechanism</u>: inhibits ergosterol synthesis by interfering with precursor assembly
2. <u>Resistance</u>: not a clinical problem
3. <u>Toxicities</u>: can cause severe hepatitis
4. <u>Cidal/static</u>: static
5. <u>Coverage</u>: used for onychomycosis (fungal toenail infection)

E. Griseofulvin

1. <u>Mechanism</u>: unclear
2. <u>Resistance</u>: can develop during prolonged therapy
3. <u>Toxicities</u>: can cause severe hepatitis, GI upset
4. <u>Cidal/static</u>: static
5. <u>Coverage</u>: used for onychomycosis (fungal toenail infection), but rarely now since terbinafine and fluconazole are available

F. Echinocandins

1. <u>Mechanism</u>: **inhibit β-1,3-glucan synthetase, a key enzyme in the synthesis of fungal cell walls**—this is the first fungal cell wall-active class of drugs
2. <u>Resistance</u>: unclear
3. <u>Toxicities</u>: virtually none
4. <u>Cidal/static</u>: cidal

5. <u>Coverage</u>: cover yeast and some molds, these drugs are a novel class, with one drug (caspofungin) FDA approved for use against *Aspergillus;* other applications still being investigated

IX. Antiparasitic Antibiotics (see Table 11.10)

A. Metronidazole

1. <u>Mechanism</u>: unknown, but may act as an electron sink, depriving organisms of necessary reducing equivalents

2. <u>Toxicities</u>: **has a disulfiram-like effect with alcohol,** can cause a metallic aftertaste

3. <u>Coverage</u>: covers GI and vaginal protozoa, especially *Entamoeba, Giardia,* and *Trichomonas*

B. Iodoquinol

1. <u>Mechanism</u>: unknown

2. <u>Toxicities</u>: iodine-related skin irritation and thyroid dysfunction—not likely to be tested on the Boards

3. <u>Coverage</u>: **used in combination with metronidazole to treat *Entamoeba,* because metronidazole does not hit the cystic forms of the protozoa but iodoquinol will**

C. Quinine derivatives

1. <u>Mechanism</u>: unknown

2. <u>Toxicities</u>: a number of toxicities have been reported, but the **testable ones are hemolysis in G6PD deficiency and retinal toxicity**

3. <u>Coverage</u>: *Plasmodium spp.*

D. Folate antagonists

1. <u>Mechanism</u>: block folate synthesis

2. <u>Toxicities</u>: allergic reactions to sulfa moieties, hemolysis in G6PD deficiency

3. <u>Coverage</u>: 1st line for *Toxoplasma* in combination with sulfadiazine; also used for *Plasmodium* and *Pneumocystis*

E. Suramin

1. <u>Mechanism</u>: unknown

2. <u>Toxicities</u>: can be severe, leading to rapid shock and death—not likely to be tested

3. <u>Coverage</u>: African *Trypanosoma*

Table 11.10 Antiparasitic Antibiotics

Drug	Characteristics
metronidazole	• Covers intestinal/hepatic amebiasis, *Giardia*, and *Trichomonas*
iodoquinol	• Kills amebic cysts, which metronidazole does not, so used in combination
chloroquine	• Used for prophylaxis and therapy of nonresistant *Plasmodium* • Resistance is increasingly common throughout the world • Monitor for retinal toxicity with prolonged use
primaquine	• The only quinine derivative that kills liver phase *P. ovale/vivax* • Used in combination with chloroquine for these species • Causes hemolysis in pts with G6PD deficiency
mefloquine	• Used as prophylaxis or treatment for chloroquine-resistant malaria • Can rarely cause psychosis, but otherwise well tolerated
quinine	• The original malaria therapy, but has the smallest therapeutic window • May be active even against malaria resistant to chloroquine & mefloquine • Adverse effects = cinchonism → tinnitus, hearing loss, GI distress
pyrimethamine	• Specific inhibitor of protozoal dihydrofolate reductase • 1st line for active *Toxoplasma* disease in combo with sulfadiazine
pyrimethamine + sulfadoxine	• Used to treat chloroquine-resistant malaria • Can cause fatal allergic reactions
trimethoprim sulfamethoxazole	• 1st line for prophylaxis of *Toxoplasma* & *Pneumocystis* in AIDS pts
suramin	• Used for African *Trypanosoma* (sleeping sickness)
nifurtimox	• Used for American *Trypanosoma* (Chagas' disease)

Table 11.10 (Continued)

Drug	Characteristics
stibogluconate	• Used for *Leishmania*
atovaquone	• 2nd-line agent for *Pneumocystis* in pts intolerant of Bactrim • Used with proguanil for prophylaxis & treatment of malaria • Used in combination with pyrimethamine for *Toxoplasma*
pentamidine	• Aerosolized form → 2nd line for *Pneumocystis* in pts intolerant of Bactrim
mebendazole	• Used for intestinal nematode infections
albendazole	• 1st line for several helminthic infections because of efficacy of single dose • Covers intestinal nematodes, *Echinococcus*, neurocysticercosis • 1st line for tapeworms and most intestinal nematodes
thiabendazole	• More toxic than mebendazole or albendazole, so use limited
pyrantel pamoate	• A depolarizing neuromuscular blocker for helminths • Paralysis of the worm allows gut expulsion • Used for intestinal nematodes
diethylcarbamazine	• Used for tissue helminths, especially elephantiasis (lymph dwellers)
ivermectin	• Broad spectrum for helminths: 1st line for *Strongyloides* & *Onchocerca*
praziquantel	• 1st-line agent for all flukes, 2nd line for tapeworms (behind albendazole)
niclosamide	• 1st line for tapeworms except *Taenia solium* due to worsening of autoinfection
nitazoxanide	• New drug, extremely broad spectrum • Approved for use against *Giardia* and *Cryptosporidium*, but also covers a variety of helminths

F. Nifurtimox
1. <u>Mechanism</u>: unclear
2. <u>Toxicities</u>: neuropathy—not likely to be tested
3. <u>Coverage</u>: Chagas' disease (American *Trypanosoma*)

G. Stibogluconate
1. <u>Mechanism</u>: unknown
2. <u>Toxicities</u>: arrhythmias—not likely to be tested
3. <u>Coverage</u>: *Leishmania*

H. Atovaquone (+ Proguanil)
1. <u>Mechanism</u>:
   (a) Atovaquone is a selective inhibitor of parasite mitochondrial electron transport
   (b) Proguanil inhibits dihydrofolate reductase in *Plasmodium spp.* (that cause malaria)
2. <u>Toxicities</u>:
   (a) Atovaquone may cause diarrhea
   (b) Atovaquone + Proguanil may cause GI upset
3. <u>Coverage</u>:
   (a) Atovaquone covers *Pneumocystis, Toxoplasma*
   (b) Atovaquone + Proguanil is extremely effective as prophylaxis or therapy against malaria

I. Pentamidine
1. <u>Mechanism</u>: unknown
2. <u>Toxicities</u>: numerous, including allergic reactions, **pancreatitis**, hypoglycemia, renal failure
3. <u>Coverage</u>: **in aerosolized form as 2nd-line agent for *Pneumocystis*** in those intolerant to trimethoprim-sulfamethoxazole

J. Benzimidazoles (mebendazole, albendazole, thiabendazole)
1. <u>Mechanism</u>: unknown
2. <u>Toxicities</u>: allergic reactions—not likely to be tested
3. <u>Coverage</u>: these agents are 1st line for intestinal nematode infections

K. Pyrantel pamoate
1. <u>Mechanism</u>: **acts as a depolarizing neuromuscular blocking agent in helminths** (the equivalent of succinylcholine for humans)
2. <u>Toxicities</u>: minimal
3. <u>Coverage</u>: used for intestinal nematodes, principally *Enterobius*

L. Diethylcarbamazine

1. Mechanism: acts as a neuromuscular blocker and also potentiates immune response to tissue helminths

2. Toxicities: tissue reactions to the dying worms—not likely to be tested

3. Coverage: used for tissue helminths, especially *Wuchereria*, *Brugia*, and *Loa loa*

M. Ivermectin

1. Mechanism: neuromuscular blocker

2. Toxicities: tissue reaction to dying worms—not likely to be tested

3. Coverage: 1st line for *Strongyloides* and *Onchocerca*, also used for lymph dwellers (e.g., *Wuchereria* and *Brugia*), *Loa loa*, scabies, and some intestinal nematodes

N. Praziquantel

1. Mechanism: **neuromuscular blocker of flatworms** (platyhelminthes)

2. Toxicities: tissue reaction to dying worms—not likely to be tested

3. Coverage: **covers almost all flatworms**, both cestodes (tapeworms) and trematodes (flukes), 1st line for *Schistosoma* and liver, lung, and intestinal flukes

O. Niclosamide

1. Mechanism: **inhibits oxidative phosphorylation** in worms

2. Toxicities: poorly absorbed so minimal toxicities

3. Coverage: used for all tapeworms, but may actually exacerbate autoinfection of *Taenia solium*, because it kills the adult but not the ova, leading to disintegration of the adult and increased release of viable ova—praziquantel thus preferred for *Taenia solium* because praziquantel does kill ova

P. Nitazoxanide

1. Mechanism: inhibition of pyruvate:ferredoxin oxidoreductase (PFOR) enzyme-dependent electron transfer reaction, which is essential to anaerobic energy metabolism

2. Toxicities: very mild, largely GI upset

3. Coverage: very broad coverage of many types of parasites; indicated for *Giardia* and *Cryptosporidium*, but demonstrated activity against a variety of helminths as well

X. Antiviral Drugs (Not Antiretrovirals) (see Table 11.11)

Table 11.11 Antiviral Drugs (Not Antiretrovirals)

Drug	Characteristics
acyclovir	• 1st line for HSV-1, HSV-2, VZV; does NOT cover CMV • Relatively nontoxic, can cause CNS toxicity in pts with renal failure
valacyclovir	• As per acyclovir, but has longer half-life so less frequent dosing required
ganciclovir	• 1st line for CMV, but causes bone marrow suppression
penciclovir	• Similar to acyclovir, but toxicities may be milder
famciclovir	• The oral prodrug of penciclovir
cidofovir	• Broad-spectrum agent, active even against viruses resistant to acyclovir
foscarnet	• Covers ganciclovir-resistant CMV, and covers HIV
idoxuridine	• Only useful as a topical agent for HSV keratitis
amantadine	• Can be used for influenza A prophylaxis in those at high risk
rimantadine	• Similar to amantadine
lamivudine	• 1st line for chronic HBV, also part of HAART therapy for HIV
ribavirin	• 1st line for RSV and HCV (with interferon-α)
zanamivir	• 1st line for influenzas A and B prophylaxis and treatment • Drug delivered via an inhaler
oseltamivir	• 1st line for influenza (both A and B) prophylaxis and treatment • Drug delivered via oral tablets
interferon-α	• Used for chronic HBV and HCV (with ribavirin)

A. Acyclovir

1. Mechanism: acyclovir is phosphorylated by herpes viral thymidine kinase to acyclovir-triphosphate, which inhibits DNA polymerase and also acts as a DNA chain terminator

2. Resistance: becoming a problem

3. Toxicities: can cause CNS toxicity → confusion, hallucination, tremor, etc., or renal failure from crystal deposition—toxicity more likely to occur in pt with underlying renal failure

4. <u>Coverage</u>: **1st line for herpes simplex virus (HSV)-1, HSV-2, and varicella-zoster virus (VZV), does not cover cytomegalovirus (CMV)**

B. Valacyclovir is similar to acyclovir but has a longer half-life, necessitating less frequent dosing

C. Ganciclovir
   1. <u>Mechanism</u>: inhibits viral DNA polymerase but does not act as a chain terminator
   2. <u>Resistance</u>: less common than acyclovir
   3. <u>Toxicities</u>: **neutropenia**, much more frequent and worse than for acyclovir
   4. <u>Coverage</u>: **1st line for CMV**

D. Penciclovir
   1. <u>Mechanism</u>: similar to acyclovir, inhibits viral DNA polymerase, but unlike acyclovir, triphosphorylated penciclovir does not lead to DNA chain termination
   2. <u>Resistance</u>: cross-resistance with acyclovir
   3. <u>Toxicities</u>: mild
   4. <u>Coverage</u>: similar to acyclovir → HSV-1, HSV-2, VZV

E. Famciclovir is a prodrug of penciclovir that can be taken orally and is converted to penciclovir in vivo

F. Cidofovir
   1. <u>Mechanism</u>: inhibits viral DNA polymerase and causes chain termination, but unlike acyclovir **cidofovir is activated by cellular phosphorylases, not viral phosphorylases**
   2. <u>Resistance</u>: unusual
   3. <u>Toxicities</u>: nephrotoxicity and neutropenia
   4. <u>Coverage</u>: **very broad-spectrum coverage**, including HSV-1, HSV-2, VZV, and does cover CMV, as well as Epstein-Barr virus (EBV) and a variety of DNA viruses (e.g., poxviruses, adenovirus, papillomavirus)

G. Foscarnet
   1. <u>Mechanism</u>: **a pyrophosphate analog that directly inhibits viral DNA polymerase or reverse transcriptase** (does not need to be activated within the cell)
   2. <u>Resistance</u>: occurs but is rare
   3. <u>Toxicities</u>: nephrotoxicity
   4. <u>Coverage</u>: **covers even ganciclovir-resistant CMV, VZV, HSV, and also covers HIV**

H. Idoxuridine
1. Mechanism: an iodinated thymidine analog that inhibits DNA replication
2. Resistance: does occur clinically
3. Toxicities: **only used topically,** causing topical allergic/irritant reactions
4. Coverage: used for HSV keratitis

I. Amantadine
1. Mechanism: **inhibits viral uncoating after entry into cell**
2. Resistance: not a major clinical problem
3. Toxicities: can cause seizures and arrhythmias at high doses
4. Coverage: shortens duration of **influenza A virus infection**

J. Rimantadine is similar to amantadine

K. Lamivudine (3TC)
1. Mechanism: **a nucleoside analog that inhibits the reverse transcriptase of both hepatitis B virus (HBV) and HIV**
2. Resistance: is expected to develop during monotherapy for either HBV or HIV
3. Toxicities: can cause hepatic failure from inhibition of mitochondrial DNA synthesis
4. Coverage: used for therapy of chronic HBV infection and as part of highly active antiretroviral therapy (HAART) for HIV

L. Ribavirin
1. Mechanism: a guanosine analog that inhibits a number of viral enzymes, thereby inhibiting RNA/DNA synthesis
2. Resistance: not clinically seen
3. Toxicities: hemolysis and bone marrow suppression
4. Coverage: **broad spectrum, 1st line for respiratory syncytial virus (RSV) in kids, 1st line in combination with interferon-α for therapy of chronic hepatitis C virus (HCV)** infection, also inhibits a variety of other viruses, including some hemorrhagic fever viruses (e.g., Lassa fever)

M. Zanamivir
1. Mechanism: **a sialic acid analog that inhibits the neuraminidase enzyme of influenza A and B viruses**
2. Resistance: not yet a problem clinically
3. Toxicities: **an inhaled drug, so may cause mild bronchospasm**
4. Coverage: **1st line for prophylaxis of influenza in close contacts of infected pts, and also shortens duration of influenza infection if started early in the course**

N. Oseltamivir
1. Mechanism: **a sialic acid analog that inhibits the neuraminidase enzyme of influenza A and B viruses**
2. Resistance: not yet a problem clinically
3. Toxicities: **orally administered so can cause mild GI upset**
4. Coverage: **1st line for prophylaxis of influenza in close contacts of infected points, and also shortens duration of influenza infection if started early in the course**

O. Interferon-α
1. Mechanism: stimulates cells in the body to resist viral infection by multiple mechanisms
2. Toxicities: recombinant interferon-α is administered subcutaneously; commonly causes severe flulike symptoms and can cause severe depression
3. Coverage: used for chronic HBV infection and with ribavirin for chronic HCV

XI. Antiretroviral Drugs (see Table 11.12)

A. Nucleoside reverse transcriptase inhibitors (NRTIs) (see Table 11.12 for individual drugs)
1. All are nucleoside analogs that are converted to nucleotides inside cells
2. **They all lack 3′ acceptor sites for incoming nucleotides, and thus all act by inhibiting DNA strand synthesis after being incorporated into the growing chain**
3. **Resistance is invariable to all of these drugs unless they are used in combination with at least two other agents**
4. All are used as part of HAART for HIV
5. See Table 11.12 for individual drugs

B. Nonnucleoside reverse transcriptase inhibitors (NNRTIs)
1. **All are allosteric, noncompetitive inhibitors of reverse transcriptase**
2. They do not bind to the nucleoside-binding site of reverse transcriptase
3. **Resistance is invariable to all of these drugs unless they are used in combination with at least two other agents**
4. All are used as part of HAART for HIV
5. See Table 11.12 for individual drugs

Table 11.12 Antiretroviral Agents

Drug	Toxicity	Comments
Nucleoside Reverse Transcriptase Inhibitors (NRTIs)		
zidovudine (AZT)	Macrocytic anemia, leukopenia, neuropathy, myositis	AZT = thymidine analog with azido group (N=N=N) in place of 3' accepting oxygen, hence the name azidothymidine (AZT)
didanosine (ddI)	Pancreatitis, neuropathy	Hydroxyurea → ↓ levels of nucleotides that compete with ddI for RT → ↑ efficacy of ddI
zalcitabine (ddC)	Neuropathy	Converted to a cytosine analog in the cell
stavudine (d4T)	Neuropathy	A thymidine analog, so may antagonize AZT
lamivudine (3TC)	Hepatitis	Can also be used for HBV
emtricitabine (FTC)	Hepatitis	Can also be used for HBV
abacavir	Severe allergic rxn	Guanosine analog
tenofovir	Renal (rare)	A nucleotide analogue (already has 1 phosphorylated group, only needs 2 more)
adefovir	Renal (rare)	Used for HBV, not HIV
Nonnucleoside Reverse Transcriptase Inhibitors (NNRTIs)		
nevirapine	Rash, hepatitis	Numerous drug interactions via p450 system
delavirdine	Rash	Numerous drug interactions via p450 system
efavirenz	Dizziness, headache	Numerous drug interactions via p450 system
Protease Inhibitors (PIs)		
saquinavir	GI upset	Numerous drug interactions via p450 system
ritonavir	GI upset, paresthesias	Numerous drug interactions via p450 system
indinavir	Nephrolithiasis	Numerous drug interactions via p450 system

Table 11.12 (Continued)

Drug	Toxicity	Comments
nelfinavir	Mild GI upset	Numerous drug interactions via p450 system
amprenavir	GI upset	Numerous drug interactions via p450 system
atazanavir	Indirect hyperbilirubinemia	Same drug interactions; advantage is much less propensity to cause hyperlipidemia/cholesterolemia
lopinavir/ritonavir	GI upset	Same drug interactions; lopinavir's levels are boosted by combining with ritonavir (inhibits p450 metabolism)
Fusion Inhibitor		
enfuvirtide (T20)	Local skin reactions	Hits drug-resistant HIV, has to be administered SQ twice daily for life

C. Protease inhibitors (PIs)

1. HIV protease chops up a large precursor viral protein into smaller proteins that compose the viral core

2. **Protease inhibitors inhibit this viral protease, thereby inhibiting synthesis of new virions**

3. **Recently, long-term side effects of these agents have been described, including a lipodystrophy syndrome clinically like Cushing's syndrome (e.g., buffalo hump, truncal obesity, hypertriglyceridemia, hyperglycemia)**

4. New concept in protease inhibitor therapy is to "boost" the level of protease inhibitors by inhibiting their metabolism—the way to do this is to combine the drug with low-dose ritonavir, thereby markedly increasing serum levels of the drug and increasing efficacy (see lopinavir/ritonavir combination)

5. See Table 11.12 for individual drugs

D. Fusion inhibitor

1. The only one currently available is enfuvirtide

2. Binds to gp41 on HIV surface, preventing interaction of gp120 with CD4 on T cell surface

3. Must be administered SQ and twice daily for life

4. Extremely expensive and difficult to take, used as salvage therapy for drug-resistant virus

12. TOXICOLOGY

I. Free Radicals

A. Free radicals contain an unshared electron and act by taking electrons from nearby functional groups—they are highly reactive

B. The functional group losing the electron then becomes equally reactive, stealing an electron from another nearby functional group, and a chain reaction is begun

C. Most free radicals in biological tissues are generated from oxygen species, often from hydroxyl (OH^-)

D. Glutathione (G-SH)

1. Glutathione protects cells from the effects of free radicals by soaking up extra electrons

2. Each glutathione molecule soaks up one extra electron, then two molecules fuse to form a glutathione dimer, thereby neutralizing both electrons:

$$G\text{-}SH + O_2^- \bullet \text{ (superoxide)} \rightarrow G\text{-}S \bullet + OH^- : G\text{-}S \bullet + G\text{-}S \bullet = G\text{-}SS\text{-}G$$

3. Glutathione also protects cells from hydrogen peroxide:

$$2\ G\text{-}SH + H_2O_2 \rightarrow G\text{-}SS\text{-}G + 2\ H_2O$$

4. However, during these reactions glutathione is used up; to keep protecting cells, glutathione must be regenerated by a reaction with NADPH via glutathione reductase:

$$G\text{-}SS\text{-}G + 2\ NADPH \rightarrow 2\ G\text{-}SH + 2\ NADP^+$$

II. Toxidromes and Antidotes (see Table 12.1)

Table 12.1 Toxidromes and Antidotes

Toxin	Characteristics
acetaminophen	• <u>Si/Sx:</u> transaminitis followed by hepatic failure (↑ PT & PTT) at 48–72 hrs, renal failure develops after liver failure
	• <u>Toxic dose:</u> 7–10 g (140 mg/kg) for acute ingestions
	• <u>Mechanism:</u> metabolized by liver to free radical, depletes glutathione in liver, then causes cell destruction

Table 12.1 (Continued)

Toxin	Characteristics
	• <u>Dx</u>: serum drug level, use published nomogram comparing level to time after ingestion to determine if drug is in the toxic range • <u>Tx</u> = *N*-acetylcysteine (regenerates glutathione) is curative, use if toxicity is indicated by nomogram, Tx must begin within 12 hrs of ingestion
anticholinergics	• <u>Si/Sx</u>: hyperthermia due to lack of sweat, dry mucous membranes, confusion, poor vision from mydriasis and cycloplegia ("hot as a hare, dry as a bone, mad as a hatter, blind as a bat") • <u>Toxic dose</u>: variable depending on agent • <u>Mechanism</u>: block acetylcholine signaling • <u>Dx</u>: clinical • <u>Tx</u>: GI decontamination with charcoal, physostigmine (inhibits anticholinesterase, ↑ cholinergic signaling) for severe toxicity
arsenic	• <u>Si/Sx</u>: acutely → GI toxicity including nausea, vomiting, diarrhea, capillary leak syndrome → hypotension, hemolysis, renal failure :: chronic toxicity → hyperkeratosis, hyperpigmentation, dermatitis, Mees lines (white horizontal stripes on fingernails), bone marrow suppression, sensory neuropathy in a stocking-glove distribution, CNS depression • <u>Toxic dose</u>: 2 mg/kg can be fatal • <u>Mechanism</u>: inhibits biochemical enzyme activity in cells • <u>Dx</u>: clinical, confirm with blood level • <u>Tx</u>: gastric lavage & dimercaprol, which chelates to arsenic in the body
barbiturate	• <u>Si/Sx</u>: respiratory depression/failure, coma, miosis • <u>Toxic dose</u>: varies • <u>Mechanism</u>: GABA-ergic CNS depressant • <u>Dx</u>: blood level • <u>Tx</u>: charcoal to prevent absorption, bicarbonate to alkalinize urine, supportive Tx (e.g., intubation for respiratory depression)
benzodiazepine	• <u>Si/Sx</u> = respiratory depression/failure and coma • <u>Toxic dose</u>: varies • <u>Mechanism</u>: GABA-ergic CNS depressant

(Continued)

Table 12.1 (Continued)

Toxin	Characteristics
	• <u>Dx</u>: blood level • <u>Tx</u>: supportive (e.g., intubation for respiratory depression), flumazenil only for acute toxicity or as a diagnostic maneuver, can precipitate seizure in chronic abusers and effects do not last long enough to act as a true antidote
β-blockers	• <u>Si/Sx</u>: bradycardia, heart block, hyperkalemia, hypoglycemia, hypotension • <u>Toxic dose</u>: varies • <u>Mechanism</u>: inhibits β-adrenergic signaling • <u>Dx</u>: clinical • <u>Tx</u>: dopamine pressor, glucagon (stimulates cAMP production, which β-blockers inhibit), IV calcium
carbon monoxide	• <u>Si/Sx</u>: dyspnea, confusion, coma, cherry-red color of skin, mucosal cyanosis • <u>Toxic dose</u>: difficult to quantitate • <u>Mechanism</u>: inhibits oxygen transport in blood and oxidative metabolism in mitochondria by displacing oxygen from hemoglobin (carbon monoxide is 210 times more avid for hemoglobin than O_2) and cytochrome oxidase • <u>Dx</u>: serum carboxy-hemoglobin level • <u>Tx</u>: 100% O_2 or hyperbaric O_2
cyanide	• <u>Si/Sx</u>: in seconds to minutes → seizures or coma, lactic acidosis, paralysis, and classic "almond-scented breath" • <u>Toxic dose</u>: ≥ 50 mg • <u>Mechanism</u>: uncouples oxidative phosphorylation in mitochondria, thus inhibiting electron transport, leading to lactic acidosis and brain injury • <u>Dx</u>: clinical (blood levels not widely available) • <u>Tx</u>: amyl or sodium nitrite (nitrites induce formation of methemoglobin, which has higher affinity for cyanide than mitochondrial cytochrome oxidase) followed by sodium thiosulfate (converts the cyanide attached to methemoglobin to thiocyanate, which can be urinated out)
digoxin	• <u>Si/Sx</u> = abnormal color vision, GI upset, supraventricular tachycardia with heart block, or bradycardia with heart block, junctional escape, etc.

Table 12.1 (Continued)

Toxin	Characteristics
	• <u>Toxic dose</u>: toxicity can occur even at "therapeutic" doses and blood levels, depends on potassium levels (hypokalemia ↑ toxicity, hyperkalemia ↓ toxicity), renal function, coingestion of other drugs • <u>Mechanism</u>: poisons Na^+/K^+ ATPase → ↑ intracellular sodium and calcium, ↓ intracellular potassium, also direct cholinomimetic effects on AV node—remember digoxin binds to the potassium-binding spot on the ATPase, so ↓ potassium levels → ↑ digoxin binding → ↑ toxicity • <u>Dx</u>: clinical, blood level useful if high (are often normal in chronic toxicity) • <u>Tx</u>: Digibind = antidigoxin Fab-antibodies
ethylene glycol	• <u>Si/Sx</u>: classic metabolic, anion gap acidosis with a serum osmolar gap,[a] check urine for calcium oxalate crystals, marked CNS depression, acute renal failure • <u>Toxic dose</u>: 5–10 mL (0.1 ml/kg) • <u>Mechanism</u>: CNS depressant (much stronger than ethanol), metabolites include glycolic acid (causes anion gap acidosis), and oxalic acid, which can precipitate as crystals in many tissues, including kidney • <u>Dx</u>: blood level, urine showing oxalate crystals • <u>Tx</u> = ethanol drip, fomepizol[b]
isopropyl alcohol	• <u>Si/Sx</u>: prominent vomiting, marked ketonemia but minimal acidosis, typically there is a minimal anion gap acidosis but there is a serum osmolar gap,[a] CNS depression, hypoglycemia • <u>Toxic dose</u>: 150 ml (2 mL/kg) • <u>Mechanism</u>: isopropyl alcohol is a GI irritant and causes an anion gap, but it is metabolized to acetone, so acidosis is minimal but ketonemia is marked • <u>Dx</u>: clinical based on ketonemia with mild acidosis, confirm by drug level • <u>Tx</u>: supportive, or dialysis for marked ingestion
lead	• <u>Si/Sx</u>: classic microcytic anemia with basophilic stippling in red cells, peripheral neuropathy (classic = foot-drop), purple or silver lead lines on gums, developmental delay in children • <u>Toxic dose</u>: typically a chronic poisoning, so difficult to quantitate

(Continued)

Table 12.1 (Continued)

Toxin	Characteristics
	• <u>Mechanism</u>: a variety of unfortunate biochemical effects • <u>Dx</u>: blood level • <u>Tx</u>: chelation with EDTA or penicillamine
mercury	• <u>Si/Sx</u>: inhalation → pneumonitis with infiltrates, chronic ingestion → intention tremor, polyneuropathy with sensory loss and paresthesias, and "erethism" = loss of memory, timidity, delirium • <u>Toxic dose:</u> >10 mg/kg can be fatal • <u>Mechanism</u>: a variety of unfortunate biochemical effects • <u>Dx</u>: blood level • <u>Tx</u>: ipecac, chelation with dimercaprol or penicillamine
methanol	• <u>Si/Sx</u>: CNS depression, anion gap metabolic acidosis with a serum osmolar gap,[a] vision changes are common, funduscopic reveals optic disk hyperemia, can lead to blindness • <u>Toxic dose:</u> >15 mL can be lethal • <u>Mechanism</u>: direct CNS depression, metabolized to formaldehyde and then formic acid → marked acidosis and ocular toxicity • <u>Dx</u>: clinical based on ingestion and acidosis with vision changes, confirm with blood level • <u>Tx</u>: ethanol drip (inhibits metabolism to formic acid), hemodialysis
opioids	• <u>Si/Sx</u>: classic triad = respiratory failure, miosis, coma • <u>Toxic dose:</u> varies by drug, remember renal failure markedly prolongs opioid half-life and can ↑ toxicity • <u>Mechanism</u>: central CNS depressant, also peripheral vasodilator • <u>Dx</u>: clinical, urine tox screen can show presence of opioids, rapid reversal of Sx with naloxone is a highly specific diagnostic maneuver • <u>Tx</u>: naloxone (Narcan), short-acting so doses must be repeated frequently
organophosphates	• <u>Si/Sx</u>: hypersecretion and hypermotility → nasal and oral secretions and diarrhea, miosis, bradycardia, heart block, tremor • <u>Toxic dose:</u> varies by agent • <u>Mechanism</u>: irreversibly block acetylcholinesterase, leading to markedly prolonged cholinergic signaling

Table 12.1 (Continued)

Toxin	Characteristics
	• <u>Dx</u>: clinical, confirm with blood level • <u>Tx</u>: atropine for acute, temporary symptom relief; pralidoxime is the only antidote, but because of "aging" of the bond between the toxin and receptor, antidote must be given quickly or it will not work
salicylate (aspirin)	• <u>Si/Sx</u>: initially see respiratory alkalosis, tinnitus, and hyperthermia, followed by anion gap metabolic acidosis with a normal serum osmolar gap[a] • <u>Toxic dose</u>: > 10 g (150 mg/kg) acutely, can be much lower for chronic ingestion • <u>Mechanism</u>: a variety of unfortunate biochemical effects, including uncoupling of oxidative phosphorylation • <u>Dx</u>: blood level • <u>Tx</u>: bicarbonate to alkalinize urine, dialysis for severe overdose or renal failure
strychnine	• <u>Si/Sx</u>: classic "pseudo-seizures," which are tonic muscular contractions appearing like grand mal seizures but pt is awake the whole time, often pt has opisthotonos and risus sardonicus (like tetanus poisoning) • <u>Toxic dose</u>: 1–2 mg/kg can be lethal • <u>Mechanism</u>: blocks glycine release in CNS because glycine is inhibitory, causes uncontrolled signaling across neural synapses • <u>Dx</u>: clinical, can confirm with blood level but not widely available • <u>Tx</u>: supportive, intubate pt and paralyze them if necessary
tricyclic antidepressants	• <u>Si/Sx</u>: mimic anticholinergic poisoning, major toxicity = arrhythmia 2° to widened QRS (>100 ms), leading to torsade de pointes • <u>Toxic dose</u>: varies by drug • <u>Mechanism</u>: have anticholinergic properties, prolong QT interval by blocking ion channels in cardiac tissue • <u>Dx</u>: clinical, EKG • <u>Tx</u>: bicarbonate drip to alkalize urine

[a]Serum osmolar gap = difference between measured serum osmoles and calculated serum osmoles (osmolality = 2[Na] + [BUN]/2.8 + [glucose]/18); this gap is present in ingestions of nonionic toxins, but charged toxins do not cause an osmolar gap.

[b]See *N Engl J Med* 1999; 340:832.

III. Controlled Substances (see Table 12.2)

Table 12.2 Scheduled Controlled Substances

	Class Characteristic	Examples
Schedule I	No accepted medical indications with high abuse potential	Heroin, marijuana, LSD
Schedule II	Accepted medical indications with high abuse potential	Opioids (e.g., morphine, codeine, hydromorphone), cocaine, amphetamine derivatives (e.g., methylphenidate)
Schedule III	Compounds containing small amounts of Schedule II drugs	Suppository forms of barbiturates
Schedule IV	Abuse potential smaller than Schedule III	Phenobarbital, benzodiazepines
Schedule V	Compounds containing limited quantities of Schedule IV drugs	Cough suppressants or antidiarrheals containing Schedule IV drugs

IV. Herbs (see Table 12.3)

Table 12.3 Herbs & Their Toxicities

Herb	Uses	Adverse Effects
chamomile	Member of the daisy family; taken as a tea for indigestion	Patients with allergies to ragweed and members of the daisy plant family should avoid these teas
chaparral (*Larrea tridentata*)	Desert shrub commonly used in traditional medicine by Native Americans; promoted as a natural antioxidant, cancer cure, and acne treatment, but evidence is scanty	Acute nonviral hepatitis, can lead to fulminant hepatic failure
echinacea	Also a member of daisy family; marketed as immune system booster, but evidence is scanty	Discouraged in pregnancy and in patients with autoimmune diseases
garlic	One of the most commonly used herbs; lowers cholesterol and is a blood thinner in large quantities;	Must be taken in very large quantities, enough to keep most people away from you

Table 12.3 (Continued)

Herb	Uses	Adverse Effects
	has antibacterial properties in vitro (no activity in vivo)	Must not be taken in conjunction with other blood thinners such as aspirin
ginger	Used for motion sickness, nausea, and indigestion	Unknown
ginkgo biloba	Studies suggest an improvement in memory and mental alertness	Excess may cause irritability and poor concentration and may inhibit platelets
ginseng	Taken as a tea to boost vitality and stamina	May cause hypertension and tachycardia
ma huang (*Ephedra*)	Similar to pseudoephedrine and amphetamine; increased energy, weight loss, and appetite suppression	Hypertension, tachycardia, prostate hypertrophy, and stroke
saw palmetto	Used to decrease prostate hypertrophy in benign prostate hypertrophy	Unknown
St. John's Wort	Used to treat depression, anxiety, and sleep disorders	Induces cytochrome p450, affecting the metabolism of many drugs such as antiretrovirals, anesthesia, analgesics, contraceptives, and antiseizure meds
willow bark (*Salix* species)	Analgesic, antirheumatic, and antipyretic properties; the same chemical properties and adverse effects as aspirin; salicin in willow bark is converted to salicylic acid by the body after ingestion.	Gastric ulcers, tinnitus, bleeding, hyperventilation, urticaria, pruritis, swelling, bronchospasms, and anaphylaxis in patients with allergy to aspirin-containing products
yohimbe (*Pausinystalia yohimbe*)	Yohimbe is a tree bark; marketed as an "enhancer of male performance and strength"; major chemical in yohimbe is yohimbine, a vasodilator; at high doses, yohimbine is a monoamine oxidase inhibitor	Incidents of renal failure, seizures, and death have been reported, and as an MAO inhibitor serious adverse effects can occur when taken concomitantly with tyramine-containing foods (e.g., liver, cheeses, red wine) or with over-the-counter nasal decongestants and diet aids

V. Teratogens

A. A teratogen is any agent that causes a fetal structural abnormality during pregnancy, resulting in the loss of the pregnancy, a birth defect, or a pregnancy complication. Teratogens include infectious agents, physical agents, maternal health factors, environmental chemicals, and drugs (see Table 12.4)

Table 12.4 Examples of Teratogens

Androgenic hormones
Angiotensin-converting enzyme inhibitors
Captopril, enalapril
Antibiotics
Tetracycline
Anticancer drugs
Aminopterin, methylaminopterin,
cyclophosphamide, busulfan
Anticonvulsants
Diphenylhydantoin, trimethadione,
valproic acid
Antithyroid drugs
Methimazole
Chelators
Penicillamine
Cocaine
Coumadin anticoagulants
Warfarin
Diethylstilbestrol
Fluconazole, high dose
Iodides
Lithium
Misoprostol
Retinoids
13-cis-retinoic acid (isotretinoin)
acitretin (Neotigason, Soriatane)
Thalidomide

B. The U.S. Food and Drug Administration (FDA) has created five drug categories to designate the safety of medications for their use during pregnancy (see Table 12.5)

Table 12.5 Current Categories for Drug Use in Pregnancy

Category	Description
A	Medication has not shown an increased risk for birth defects in human studies.
B	Animal studies have not demonstrated a risk and there are no adequate studies in humans, OR animal studies have shown a risk, but the risk has not been seen in humans.
C	Animal studies have shown adverse effects, but no studies are available in humans, OR studies in humans and animals are not available.
D	Medications that are associated with birth defects in humans; however, there may be potential benefits in rare cases that outweigh their known risks.
X	Medications are contraindicated (should not be used) in human pregnancy, because of known fetal abnormalities that have been demonstrated in both human and animal studies.

U.S. Food and Drug Administration. *FDA Consumer,* vol. 35, no. 3, May–June 2001, *online version.*

APPENDIX: COMMONLY PRESCRIBED DRUGS

Generic Drug Name	Brand Name
Abacavir	Ziagen
Abciximab	ReoPro
Acarbose	Orecise
Acetaminophen	Tylenol
Acetaminophen w/ codeine	Tylenol w/ codeine
Acetaminophen w/ oxycodone	Percocet, Tylox
Acetaminophen w/ propoxyphrene-N	Darvocet-N
Acetazolamide	Diamox
Acetylcysteine	Mucomyst
Acyclovir	Zovirax
Adefovir	Hepsera
Adenosine	Adenocard
Albendazole	Albenza
Albuterol	Proventil
Albuterol w/ ipratropium	Combivent
Alendronate	Fosamax
Allopurinol	Zyloprim
Almotriptan	Axert
Alprazolam	Xanax
Alprostadil	Caverject, Muse
Alteplase	Activase, Cathflo, t-PA
Amantadine	Symmetrel
Amikacin	Amikin
Amiloride	Midamor
Aminocaproic acid	Amicar
Amiodarone	Cordarone, Pacerone
Amitriptyline	Elavil
Amlodine	Norvasc
Amoxicillin	Amoxil, Trimox
Amoxicillin w/ potassium clavulanate	Augmentin
Amphotericin B, deoxycholate	Fungizone
Amphotericin B, lipid complex	Abelcet
Amphotericin B, liposomal	AmBisome
Ampicillin	Principen

Generic Drug Name	Brand Name
Ampicillin-sulbactam	Unasyn
Amprenavir	Agenerase
Anagrelide	Agrylin
Aprepitant	Emend
Aprotinin	Trasylol
Aripiprazole	Abilify
Asparaginase	Elspar
Aspirin, enteric-coated	ECASA
Atazanavir	Reyataz
Atenolol	Tenormin
Atomoxetine	Strattera
Atorvastatin	Lipitor
Atovaquone	Mepron
Atovaquone + proguanil	Malarone
Azacitidine	Vidaza
Azatadine	Optimine
Azathioprine	Azasan, Imuran
Azithromycin	Zithromax
Aztreonam	Azactam
Baclofen	Lioresal
Benazepril	Lotensin
Benztropine	Cogentin
Betaxolol	Kerlone
Bethanechol	Urecholine
Bisacodyl	Correctol, Dulcolax
Bismuth subsalicylate	Kaopectate, Pepto-Bismol
Bisoprolol	Zebeta
Bivalirudin	Angiomax
Bleomycin	Blenoxane
Bortezomib	Velcade
Bromocriptine	Parlodel
Budesonide	Rhinocort Aqua
Bumetanide	Bumex
Bupropion	Wellbutrin
Buspirone	Buspar
Busulfan	Myleran
Cabergoline	Dostinex
Candesartan	Atacand
Capecitabine	Xeloda
Captopril	Capoten
Carbamazepine	Tegretol
Carboplatin	Paraplatin

Generic Drug Name	Brand Name
Carisoprodol	Soma
Carmustine	Neosar
Carvedilol	Coreg
Caspofungin	Cancidas
Cefazolin	Ancef
Cefepime	Maxipime
Cefotaxime	Claforan
Ceftazidime	Cetaz, Fortaz, Tazicef, Tazidime
Ceftizoxime	Cefizox
Ceftriaxone	Rocephin
Cefuroxime	Ceftin
Celecoxib	Celebrex
Cephalexin	Keflex
Cetirizine	Zyrtec
Chlorambucil	Leukeran
Chloramphenicol	Cloromycetin
Chlordiazepoxide	Librium
Chloroquine	Aralen
Chlorpromazine	Thorazine
Chlorpropamide	Diabinese
Cholestyramine	Questran
Cidofovir	Vistide
Cimetidine	Tagamet
Cincalcet	Sensipar
Ciprofloxacin	Cipro
Cisplatin	Platinol-AQ
Citalopram	Celexa
Clarithromycin	Biaxin
Clindamycin	Cleocin
Clomiphene	Clomid, Serophene
Clonazepam	Klonopin
Clonidine	Catapress
Clopidogrel	Plavix
Clozapine	Clozaril
Colestipol	Colestid
Cromolyn sodium	Crolom
Cyclobenzaprine	Flexaril
Cyclopentolate	Cyclogyl
Cyclophosphamide	Cytoxan
Cyclosporin	Neoral, Sandimmune
Cyproheptadine	Periactin

Generic Drug Name

Generic Drug Name	Brand Name
Cytarabine	CytosarU, Tarabine
Danrolene	Dantrium
Daptomycin	Cubicin
Darbopoeitin	Aranesp
Daunorubicin	Cerbudine, DanuoXome
Desipramine	Norpramin
Desloratadine	Clarinex
Desmopressin	Stimate
Dexamethasone	Decadron
Diazapam	Valium
Dicloxacillin	Dynapen
Didanosine	Videx
Digoxin	Lanoxin
Dihydroergotamine	Migranal
Diltiazem	Cardizem, Tiazac
Dimenhydrinate	Dramamine
Diphenhydramine	Benadryl
Diphenoxylate + atropine	Lomotil
Divalproex sodium	Depakote
Dobutamine	Dobutrex
Docetaxel	Taxotere
Docusate sodium	Colace
Donepezil	Aricept
Dopamine	Intropin
Doxazosin	Cardura
Doxepin	Sinequan
Droperidol	Inapsine
Drotrecogin alpha	Xigris
Duloxetine	Cymbalta
Edrophonium	Tensilon
Efavirenz	Sustiva
Enalapril	Vasotec
Enfuvirtide	Fuzeon
Enoxaparin	Lovenox
Entacapone	Comtan
Eplerenone	Inspra
Eprosartan	Teveten
Ertapenem	Invanz
Erythropoeitin	Epogen, Procrit
Escitalopram	Lexapro
Esmolol	Brevibloc
Esomeprazole	Nexium

Generic Drug Name	Brand Name
Estrogens, conjugated	Premarin (tablets)
Estrogens, conjugated, w/ medroxyprogesterone	Prempro
Etanercept	Enbrel
Ethinyl estradiol w/ norgestimate	Ortho Tri-cyclen
Ethosuximide	Zarontin
Etomidate	Amidate
Etoposide	Etopophos, Toposar, VP16
Ezetimibe	Ezetimibe
Famciclovir	Famvir
Famotidine	Pepcid
Felbamate	Felbatol
Felodipine	Plendil
Fenofibrate	Tricor
Fentanyl	Duragesic
Fexofenadine	Allegra
Filgrastim	Neupogen
Finasteride	Proscar
Fluconazole	Diflucan
Flumazenil	Romazicon
Fluorouracil	Adrucil
Fluoxetine	Prozac
Fluphenazine	Prolixin
Flurazepam	Dalmane
Flutamide	Eulexin
Fluticasone	Flovent
Fluvastatin	Lescol
Fomepizole	Antizol
Fondaparinux	Arixtra
Foscarnet	Foscavir
Fosinopril	Monopril
Furosemide	Lasix
Gabapentin	Neurontin
Galantamine	Reminyl
Ganciclovir	Cytovene
Gatifloxacin	Tequin
Gemfibrozil	Lopid
Gentamicin	Garamycin
Glatiramer	Copaxone
Glimepiride	Amaryl
Glipizide	Glucatrol
Glyburide	Diabeta, Miconase

Generic Drug Name	Brand Name
Granisetron	Kytril
Guaifenesin	Robitussin
Haloperidol	Haldol
Hydralazine	Apresoline
Hydromorphone	Dilaudid
Hydroxyurea	Hydrea
Hydroxyzine	Ataraz, Vistaril
Ibandronate	Boniva
Ibuprofen	Advil, Motrin
Imatinib mesylate	Gleevec
Imipenem-cilastatin	Primaxin
Imipramine	Tofranil
Indinavir	Crixivan
Infliximab	Remicade
Insulin glargine	Lantus
Insulin isophane, human recombinant	Humulin N
Insulin lispro	Humalog
Insulin regular w/ isophane, human recombinant	Humulin 70/30
Interferon alpha	Infergen, Intron A
Interferon beta	Avonex, Betaseron
Ipratropium	Atrovent
Isoretinoin	Accutane
Isosorbide dinitrate	Isordile
Itraconazole	Sporanox
Ketamine	Ketalar
Ketoconazole	Nizoral
Labetalol	Normodyne, Trandate
Lactulose	Chronulac
Lamivudine	Epivir
Lamotrigine	Lamictal
Lansoprazole	Prevacid
Latanoprost	Xalatan
Leflunomide	Arava
Levetiracetam	Keppra
Levodopa-carbidopa	Atamet, Sinemet
Levofloxacin	Levaquin
Levothyroxine	Synthroid
Lidocaine	Lidoderm, Xylocaine
Linezolid	Zyvox
Lisinopril	Prinivil, Zestril

Generic Drug Name	Brand Name
Lithium	Carbolith, Duralith, Eskalith, Lithobid
Loperamide	Imodium
Lopinavir-ritonavir	Kaletra
Loratadine	Claritin
Lorazepam	Ativan
Losartan	Cozaar
Meclizine HCL	Antivert
Medroxyprogesterone	Provera
Mefloquine	Lariam
Megestrol	Megace
Memantine	Namenda
Meperidine	Demerol
Meropenem	Merrem
Metformin	Glucophage
Methyldopa	Aldomet
Methylprednisolone	Medrol
Metoclopramide	Reglan
Metoprolol	Lopressor
Metronidazole	Flagyl
Micafungin	Mycamine
Midazolam	Versed
Milrinone	Primacor
Minocycline	Minocin
Minoxidil	Loniten
Mometasone	Nasonex
Montelukast	Singulair
Moxifloxacin	Avelox
Mupirocin	Bactroban
Mycophenolate mofetil	Cellcept
Naloxone	Narcan
Naproxen	Anaprox, Naprosyn
Nelfinavir	Viracept
Neostigmine	Prostigmin
Nesiritide	Natrecor
Nevirapine	Viramune
Nifedipine	Adalat
Nimodipine	Nimotop
Nitrofurantoin	Macrobid, Macrodantin
Nitroprusside	Nipride, Nitropress
Nizatidine	Axid
Norepinephrine	Levophed

Generic Drug Name	Brand Name
Nortriptyline	Aventyl
Nystatin	Mycostatin
Octreotide	Sandostatin
Olanzapine	Zyprexa
Omeprazole	Prilosec
Ondansetron	Zofran
Orlistat	Xenical
Oseltamivir	Tamiflu
Oxacillin	Bactocill
Oxybutynin chloride	Ditropan
Oxycodone	OxyContin
Oxymetazoline	Afrin
Pamidronate	Aredia
Pantoprazole	Protonix
Paroxetine	Paxil
Peg-filgrastim	Neulasta
Peg-interferon alpha	Pegasys, PEG-Intron
Pentobarbital	Nembutal
Pentoxifylline	Trental
Pergolide	Permax
Phenazopyridine HCL	Pyridium
Phenelzine	Nardil
Phenoxybenzamine	Dibenzyline
Phentolamine	Regitine, Rogitine
Phenylephrine	Neo-Synephrine
Phenytoin	Dilantin
Pilocarpine	Pilocar
Pimecrolimus	Elidel
Pioglitazone	Actos
Piperacillin	Pipracil
Piperacillin-tazobactam	Zosyn
Pralidozime	Protopam
Pramipexole	Mirapex
Pravastatin	Pravachol
Prazosin	Minipress
Procainamide	Procanbid, Pronestyl
Prochlorperazine	Compazine
Promethazine	Phenergan
Propofol	Diprivan
Propranolol	Inderal
Pseudoephedrine	Sudafed
Psyllium	Fiberall, Metamucil

Generic Drug Name	Brand Name
Pyridostigmine	Mestinon, Regonal
Quetiapine	Seroquel
Quinapril	Accupril
Rabeprazole	AcipHex
Raloxifene	Evista
Ramipril	Altace
Ranitidine	Zantac
Repaglinide	Prandin
Ribavirin	Rebetol, Virazole
Rimantidine	Flumadine
Risedronate	Actonel
Risperidone	Risperdal
Ritonavir	Norvir
Rituximab	Rituxan
Rivastigmine	Exelon
Rocuronium	Zemuron
Ropinirole	Requip
Rosiglitazone	Avandia
Rosuvastatin	Crestor
Salmeterol	Serevent
Scopolamine	Transderm-Scop
Selegiline	Eldepryl
Senna	Senokot
Sertraline	Zoloft
Sildenafil	Viagra
Simethicone	Gas-X, Mylicon, Phazyme
Simvastatin	Zocor
Sotalol	Betapace
Spironolactone	Aldactone
Stavudine (d4T)	Zerit
Sucralfate	Carafte
Sumatriptan	Imitrex
Tacrolimus	Prograf
Tadalafil	Cialis
Tamoxifen	Nolvadex
Tegaserod	Zelnorm
Telithromycin	Ketek
Temazepam	Restoril
Tenecteplase	TNKase
Tenofovir (TDF)	Viread
Terazosin	Hytrin
Terbinafine	Lamisil

Generic Drug Name	Brand Name
Theophylline	Elixophyllin, Theo-Dur, Uniphyl
Thiopental	Pentothal
Ticarcillin	Ticar
Ticarcillin-clavulanate	Timentin
Tinzaparin	Innohep
Tiotropium	Spiriva
Tirofiban	Aggrastat
Tizanidine	Zanaflex
Tolcapone	Tasmar
Tolterodine	Detrol
Topiramate	Topamax
Tramadol	Ultram
Trazodone	Desyrel
Tretinoin	Renova, Retin-A
Triamcinolone (inhaled)	Azmacort
Triamcinolone w/ acetonide (nasal)	Nasacort AQ
Triamcinolone w/ acetonide (topical)	Kenalog
Triazolam	Halcion
Trihexyphenidyl	Artane
Trimethobenzamide	Tigan
Trimethoprim-sulfamethoxazole	Bactrim, Septra
Valacyclovir	Valtrex
Valdecoxib	Bextra
Valganciclovir	Valcyte
Valproic acid	Depakene, Depakote
Valsartan	Diovan
Vancomycin	Vancocin
Vardenafil	Levitra
Vasopressin	Pitressin
Vecuronium	Norcuron
Venlafaxine	Effexor
Verapamil	Calan
Voriconazole	V-fend
Warfarin	Coumadin
Zafirlukast	Accolate
Zanamivir	Relenza
Zidovudine (AZT)	Retrovir
Ziprasidone	Geodon
Zoledronic acid	Zometa
Zolpidem	Ambien

REVIEW QUESTIONS

$$R-CH_2-NH_2 \underset{-H^+}{\overset{+H^+}{\rightleftharpoons}} R-CH_2-NH_3^+ \, (pK_a = 9.4)$$

1. A drug like that illustrated above is administered orally to a patient. Which of the following statements is correct?
   A. over 50% of the drug will accumulate in the stomach
   B. about 50% of the drug will be ionized in the plasma
   C. about 50% of the drug will be un-ionized in the stomach
   D. the drug will not be ion-trapped in acidic urine
   E. alkalinization of the urine will accelerate elimination of the drug

2. An acidic drug with a pK_a of 7.4 will:
   A. exist 50% in the ionized form in plasma
   B. be absorbed more easily from the small intestine than from the stomach
   C. be eliminated more slowly after alkalinization of the urine
   D. accumulate in stomach contents

3. Some drugs can be classified as "partial agonists." A partial agonist differs from a "full agonist" in that:
   A. the partial agonist occupies fewer receptors than does the full agonist at equivalent effective doses
   B. the partial agonist is usually less potent than the full agonist
   C. partial agonists act as antagonists in addition to acting as agonists for the same receptor type
   D. the partial agonist is usually more rapidly metabolized than is the full agonist
   E. partial agonists must be administered by IV injection

4. All of the following statements are true EXCEPT:
   A. competitive antagonists reduce the potency of the true agonist
   B. competitive antagonists reduce the efficacy of the true agonist
   C. irreversible antagonists reduce the efficacy of the true agonist
   D. partial agonists often have identical potencies but reduced efficacies compared to the true agonist

5. Intravenous drug testing in patients reveals that Drug A has a volume of distribution of 20 L/kg, whereas Drug B has a volume of distribution of 0.01 L/kg. If both drugs are given in equal doses IV, which of the following is true?

A. Drug A is more rapidly metabolized than is Drug B
B. Drug A is more rapidly absorbed from the intestine than is Drug B
C. both a and b are true
D. Drug A is tightly bound to plasma proteins
E. the plasma concentration immediately after administration of Drug A is much lower than the plasma concentration immediately after administration of Drug B

6. Antagonism of D_2-receptors and agonism of 5-HT_4 receptors results in:

A. inhibition of emesis
B. effective treatment of motion sickness
C. decreased gastric acid production
D. prolonged gastric-emptying time
E. effective treatment of gastric ulcers

7. Inhibition of neuronal release of norepinephrine can be caused by administration of which of the following drugs?

A. phentolamine
B. prazosin
C. tyramine
D. cocaine
E. clonidine

8. Early symptoms of salicylate toxicity include all of the following EXCEPT:

A. respiratory alkalosis
B. respiratory acidosis
C. tinnitus
D. anion gap metabolic acidosis
E. hyperventilation

9. Which of the following drugs releases both FSH and LH only when given in a pulsatile form?

A. cyproheptadine
B. lovastatin
C. GnRH
D. human chorionic gonadotropin
E. growth hormone

10. Which of the following drugs is the most potent in causing sodium retention?

A. hydrocortisone
B. prednisolone
C. betamethasone

    D. dexamethasone

    E. triamcinolone

11. Dexamethasone can cause all of the following side effects EXCEPT:

    A. peptic ulcers

    B. hypoglycemia

    C. osteoporosis

    D. necrosis of the femoral head

    E. personality or mood changes

12. Which of the following drugs causes the most prolonged hypoglycemic state?

    A. glyburide

    B. glipizide

    C. metformin

    D. pioglitazone

    E. chlorpropamide

13. Which of the following drugs works by inducing expression of insulin receptors and inhibiting gluconeogenesis?

    A. pioglitazone

    B. glipizide

    C. metformin

    D. chlorpropamide

    E. acarbose

14. Match the following case scenarios with the drugs most associated with them:

    A. a diabetic newly started on this drug is admitted to the hospital three weeks later in severe congestive heart failure

    B. a patient complains of abdominal distention and flatulence

    C. a patient complains of 15-pound weight gain

    D. you recommend this drug be with held in a patient scheduled to undergo a CT of the abdomen with contrast

    1. arabose

    2. metformin

    3. glipizone

    4. rosiglitazone

15. What two patient characteristics make metformin an ideal drug? (Pick two answers)

    A. pt is obese

    B. pt has renal failure

   C. pt is hypertensive as well as diabetic
   D. pt has a history of hypoglycemia on other agents
   E. pt has heart failure

16. Digoxin can cause all of the following adverse effects EXCEPT:

   A. arrhythmias
   B. sinus bradycardia
   C. vomiting
   D. visual problems
   E. rapid response atrial fibrillation

17. Which of the following antimicrobial drugs is effective against infections caused by *Bacteroides fragilis*?

   A. cefamandole
   B. cefotaxime
   C. cefotetan
   D. cefazolin
   E. cephalexin

18. Which of the following drugs is the most effective for treating infections caused by *Toxoplasma gondii*?

   A. pentamidine
   B. primaquine
   C. sodium stibogluconate
   D. pyrimethamine and sulfadiazine
   E. paromomycin

19. Which of the following aminoglycosides is often effective against organisms resistant to gentamicin?

   A. tobramycin
   B. streptomycin
   C. amikacin
   D. neomycin

20. Which of the following drugs has NO activity against anaerobes?

   A. clindamycin
   B. gentamicin
   C. metronidazole
   D. chloramphenicol
   E. penicillin G

For questions 21–23, refer to the following case presentation:
A 50-year-old male with a 30-pack-year history of smoking and alcohol abuse presents with a softball-sized mass protruding up from his lower mandible and a fever of 101°F (38.3°C). Purulent-looking material is draining from the surface of the mass. Suspecting a squamous cell head and neck cancer, you admit the patient for IV antibiotics and

nutrition. You start the patient on clindamycin for the superinfection, and he defervesces. Three days later he suddenly spikes to 102°F (38.8°C) and develops fulminant, severe diarrhea and abdominal pain. There is no rebound on exam, and the patient has hyperactive bowel sounds.

21. What is your diagnosis?
    A. paraneoplastic syndrome
    B. acute surgical abdomen
    C. malingering
    D. *Clostridium difficile* colitis
    E. metastases of the tumor to the bowel

22. What is your initial management?
    A. stop the clindamycin and give IV fluids
    B. broaden bacterial coverage by adding gentamicin and ampicillin for better bowel flora coverage
    C. continue therapy until results of stool studies return
    D. stop the parenteral nutrition and begin enteral feeding

23. What antibiotic is most appropriate to treat this process?
    A. vancomycin IV
    B. clindamycin PO
    C. ampicillin/sulbactam IV
    D. metronidazole IV or PO
    E. no antibiotic should be given

24. Isoniazid causes a peripheral neuropathy by causing deficiency of which of the following?
    A. thiamine (vitamin B_1)
    B. riboflavin (vitamin B_2)
    C. pyridoxine (vitamin B_6)
    D. cobalamin (vitamin B_{12})
    E. niacin

25. Which of the following antiviral drugs depends on virus-encoded thymidine kinase for initial phosphorylation?
    A. idoxuridine
    B. cidofovir
    C. foscarnet
    D. cytarabine
    E. acyclovir

26. Which of the following drugs does NOT cause peripheral neuropathy?
    A. didanosine (ddI)
    B. zalcitabine (ddC)

C. vincristine
D. vinblastine
E. isoniazid

27. Which of the following drugs is not nephrotoxic?
    A. gentamicin
    B. vancomycin
    C. amphotericin B
    D. clarithromycin
    E. cisplatin

28. All of the following drugs affect the microtubule system EXCEPT:
    A. paclitaxel
    B. vincristine
    C. colchicine
    D. tamoxifen

29. Metronidazole is effective in treating all of the following infections EXCEPT:
    A. amebiasis
    B. anaerobic bacteria
    C. methicillin-resistant *Staphylococcus* infections
    D. trichomoniasis
    E. giardiasis

30. Which of the following is useful to eradicate hepatic stages of malaria infection?
    A. chloroquine
    B. quinine
    C. primaquine
    D. antifolate drugs
    E. mefloquine

Questions 31–34 refer to the following list of drugs:
A. sodium iodide
B. propylthiouracil
C. propranolol
D. radioactive iodine

31. Which drug should be given FIRST to a patient with thyroid storm?

32. Which drug acts MOST rapidly to inhibit T4 release from the thyroid?

33. Which drug can INCREASE T4 release from the thyroid?

34. Which drug should be given SECOND to a patient with thyroid storm?

Questions 35–36 refer to the following list of drugs:
A. metoclopramide
B. kaolin
C. loperamide
D. magnesium hydroxide
E. omeprazole

35. Which of the preceding drugs treats diarrhea by interacting with specific receptors in the GI tract?

36. Which of the preceding drugs is useful to treat constipation?

Questions 37–39 refer to the following list of drugs:
A. nitrous oxide
B. halothane
C. succinylcholine
D. fentanyl
E. ketamine

37. Which of the preceding drug produces unconsciousness, analgesia, and amnesia at doses that do not cause cardiovascular depression?

38. Which of the preceding drugs produces neuroleptanalgesia when administered together with antipsychotic agents?

39. Which of the preceding drugs can lead to dangerous hyperkalemia in patients with crush injuries?

Questions 40–43 refer to the following list of drugs:
A. cholestyramine
B. lovastatin
C. gemfibrozil
D. clofibrate
E. niacin

40. Which of these drugs inhibits the rate-limiting step in cholesterol synthesis?

41. Which of the preceding drugs, when used in combination with lovastatin, often causes skeletal muscle pain?

42. Which of the preceding drugs most effectively lowers triglyceride levels?

43. Which of the preceding drugs increases 7-hydroxylase-mediated breakdown of cholesterol?

Questions 44–46 refer to the following list of drugs:

A. diphenhydramine
B. phenelzine
C. L-dopa
D. bromocriptine
E. deprenyl

44. Which of the preceding drugs should not be taken while the patient is eating cheeses and drinking wine?

45. Which of the preceding drugs inhibits prolactin secretion?

46. Dyskinesias are associated with chronic therapy of which of the preceding drugs?

Questions 47–49 refer to the following list of drugs:

A. phencyclidine
B. cannabis
C. cocaine
D. LSD
E. heroin

47. Which of the preceding drugs can cause long-lasting psychotic episodes?

48. Which of the preceding drugs can cause sensory inversion?

49. Which of the preceding drugs causes "pinpoint pupils"?

Questions 50–52 refer to the following list of drugs:

A. ondansetron
B. metoclopramide
C. sumatriptan
D. cisapride
E. buspirone

50. Which of the preceding drugs works as an anti-emetic by blocking dopamine receptors?

51. Which of the preceding drugs works as an anti-emetic by blocking $5\text{-}HT_3$ receptors?

52. Activation of $5\text{-}HT_1$ receptors by which of the preceding drugs causes an anxiolytic effect?

Questions 53–57 refer to the following list of drugs:

A. ipratropium bromide
B. albuterol

C. triamcinolone
D. cromolyn sodium
E. theophylline

53. Which of the preceding drugs inhibits vagally mediated bronchoconstriction?

54. Which of the preceding drugs most effectively decreases airway inflammation in chronic, recurrent asthmatics?

55. Which of the preceding drugs is the most effective bronchodilator for asthmatics?

56. Which of the preceding drugs has a narrow therapeutic index and can cause seizures at therapeutic doses?

57. Which of the preceding drugs stabilizes mast cell membranes?

Questions 58–61 refer to the following list of drugs:
A. furosemide
B. hydrochlorothiazide
C. spironolactone
D. acetazolamide

58. Which of the preceding drugs is a 1st-line antihypertensive agent?

59. Which of the preceding drugs decreases mortality in patients with heart failure?

60. Which of the preceding drugs causes a bicarbonate-wasting metabolic acidosis?

61. Which of the preceding drugs is the most effective diuretic for maintaining water loss in patients with heart failure?

62. Match the following diseases with 1st-line drugs (drugs can be used more than once):

A. essential hypertension	**1.** β-blockers
B. diabetic hypertensive pt	**2.** ACE inhibitors
C. postmyocardial infarction pt	**3.** thiazide diuretic
D. hypertensive pt with BPH	**4.** α-blockers
E. hypertensive pt with osteoporosis	**5.** spironolactone
F. proteinuria	**6.** HMG-CoA reductase
G. heart failure	inhibitors

Questions 63–67 refer to the following list of drugs:
A. melphalan
B. bleomycin

C. cisplatin
D. doxorubicin
E. methotrexate
F. imatinib mesylate

63. Which of the preceding drugs promotes DNA interstrand cross-linking and causes bone marrow suppression and alopecia but no renal or bladder toxicity?

64. Which of the preceding drugs causes prominent pulmonary fibrosis?

65. Which of the preceding drugs causes severe renal failure and emesis without much bone marrow suppression?

66. Which of the preceding drugs causes dilated cardiomyopathy?

67. Which of the preceding drugs was developed as a result of targeted drug design, based on the biology of a cancer cell?

Questions 68–70 refer to the following list of drugs:
A. methotrexate
B. cytarabine
C. 6-mercaptopurine
D. 6-thioguanine
E. carmustine

68. Leucovorin is used to rescue patients from the toxicity caused by which of the preceding drugs?

69. Allopurinol can enhance the toxicity of which of the preceding drugs?

70. Which drug is particularly lipophilic, making it useful to treat CNS tumors?

Questions 71–75 refer to the following list of drugs:
A. sulfasalazine
B. ceftazidime
C. trimethoprim
D. amoxicillin
E. oxacillin

71. Which of the preceding drugs inhibits dihydrofolate reductase?

72. Which of the preceding drugs is especially designed to treat *Staphylococcus aureus* infection?

73. Which of the preceding drugs is not well absorbed orally and is therefore used to treat bowel inflammatory disorders?

74. Which of the preceding drugs is designed to treat nosocomial gram-negative rod infections, especially *Pseudomonas*?

75. Which of the preceding drugs is highly orally absorbed?

Questions 76–80 refer to the following list of drugs:

A. vancomycin
B. aztreonam
C. cilastatin
D. levofloxacin
E. ceftriaxone

76. Which of the preceding drugs is 1st line for treating meningitis?

77. Which of the preceding drugs inhibits renal dihydropeptidase?

78. Which of the preceding drugs is only active against aerobic gram-negative rods?

79. Which of the preceding *c. difficile* drugs has essentially no oral bioavailability?

80. Which of the preceding drugs achieves essentially identical serum levels whether dosed IV or orally?

Questions 81–86 refer to the following list of drugs:

A. erythromycin
B. rifampin
C. chloramphenicol
D. doxycycline
E. gentamicin

81. Which of the preceding drugs causes gray-baby syndrome in premature neonates?

82. Which of the preceding drugs commonly causes photosensitivity reactions?

83. Which of the preceding drugs has no gram-positive activity by itself, but synergizes with cell-wall inhibitors to provide extra killing of gram-positive organisms?

84. Which of the preceding drugs has extremely broad-spectrum activity but is rarely used as single therapy because of the high rate of resistance developing?

85. Which of the preceding drugs can cause marked GI intolerance?

86. Which of the preceding drugs can cause idiosyncratic aplastic anemia?

Questions 87–90 refer to the following list of drugs:

A. ethambutol
B. rifampin
C. pyrazinamide
D. isoniazid
E. vancomycin

87. Which of the preceding drugs can cause drug-induced lupus?

88. Which of the preceding drugs can cause optic neuritis?

89. Which of the preceding drugs routinely causes orange discoloration of body fluids?

90. Which of the preceding drugs can cause marked facial flushing, shortness of breath, and erythematous rash during infusion (the so-called "red man syndrome")?

Questions 91–95 refer to the following list of drugs:

A. nevirapine
B. didanosine (ddI)
C. stavudine (d4T)
D. lamivudine (3TC)
E. indinavir

91. Which of the preceding drugs causes nephrolithiasis?

92. Which of the preceding drugs is active against both hepatitis B and HIV?

93. Which of the preceding drugs antagonizes AZT therapy?

94. Which of the preceding drugs causes severe hepatitis?

95. The efficacy of which of the preceding drugs is markedly increased in the presence of hydroxyurea?

96. Match the following drugs with their mechanism of action:

A. ampicillin	**1.**	binds 50S ribosome, blocks
B. vancomycin		peptidyltransferase reaction
C. amikacin	**2.**	neuromuscular blocker
D. tetracycline	**3.**	blocks RNA polymerase
E. chloramphenicol	**4.**	inhibits β1-3 glucan synthesis,
F. clarithromycin		blocking cell wall formation
G. clindamycin	**5.**	binds 50S ribosome, prevents
H. linezolid		union of 50S and 30S subunits
I. ofloxacin	**6.**	blocks DNA gyrase (topoisomerase)
J. rifampin	**7.**	inhibits transpepti dase
K. amphotericin		cross-linking of peptidoglycan
L. fluconazole	**8.**	binds to 30S ribosome, causes
M. caspofungin		misreading of mRNA code
N. praziquantel	**9.**	inhibits synthesis of ergosterol
O. niclosamide	**10.**	binds to 30S ribosome, blocks
		aminoacyl-tRNA acceptor site
	11.	inhibits insertion of D-alanine-D-alanine subunits into cell wall
	12.	binds ergosterol, creating pores in cell membrane
	13.	binds 50S ribosome, blocks amino acid translocation
	14.	inhibits oxidative phosphorylation
	15.	binds 50S ribosome, blocks formation of peptide bond

Questions 97–101 refer to the following list of drugs:

A. all-trans retinoic acid
B. rituximab
C. gemtuzumab
D. interferon-α
E. imatinib mesylate
F. trastuzumab
G. G-CSF

97. Which of the preceding therapies are monoclonal antibodies (choose as many as apply)?

98. Which of the preceding therapies supports production of granulocytes in neutropenic patients?

99. Which of the preceding therapies is an enzyme inhibitor?

100. Which of the preceding therapies induces differentiation of malignant cells?

101. Which of the preceding therapies are used to treat hematologic malignant cells (choose as many as apply)?

Questions 102–109 refer to the following list of drugs:
  A. *N*-acetylcysteine
  B. Digibind
  C. pralidoxime
  D. mesna
  E. nitrite
  F. naloxone
  G. dimercaprol
  H. diphenhydramine

102. Which of the preceding compounds is given for opiate overdose?

103. Which of the preceding compounds should be immediately administered IV to a patient having a dystonic reaction to a dopamine antagonist (e.g., neuroleptic or antiemetic)?

104. Which of the preceding compounds is a chelating agent that can be used in heavy metal poisoning?

105. Which of the preceding compounds is an antidote for organophosphate poisoning?

106. Which of the preceding compounds would you use to treat junctional tachycardia in a patient in congestive heart failure on several heart failure medicines?

107. Which of the preceding compounds is an antidote for acetaminophen overdose?

108. Which of the preceding compounds is used to prevent hemorrhagic cystitis?

109. Which of the preceding compounds is used as part of a regimen to treat cyanide poisoning?

Questions 110–116 refer to the following list of drugs:
  A. epinephrine
  B. norepinephrine
  C. phenylephrine
  D. dopamine
  E. dobutamine
  F. vasopressin
  G. digoxin

110. Which of the preceding drugs is the standard 1st-line pressor for most hypotensive patients and can also promote diuresis at low doses?

111. Which of the preceding pressors is particularly useful in patients with low systemic vascular resistance (e.g., sepsis), but can promote severe tachycardia?

112. Which of the preceding pressors is particularly useful in patients who are already tachycardic?

113. Which of the preceding pressors is 1st line for cardiogenic shock, but may lower blood pressure and therefore is often combined with a second agent?

114. Which of the preceding pressors is 1st line for any pulseless patient during cardiac resuscitation?

115. Which of the preceding pressors causes minimal increase in myocardial oxygen demand?

116. Which of the preceding pressors is now considered a 1st-line option for pulseless ventricular fibrillation or tachycardia during cardiac resuscitation, but is not on the ACLS guidelines for any other type of code?

For the following questions, select which is greater, A or B.

117. **A.** Efficacy of bethanechol as a topical preparation for glaucoma
B. Efficacy of pilocarpine as a topical preparation for glaucoma

118. **A.** Magnitude of bronchoconstriction in asthmatic caused by propranolol
B. Magnitude of bronchoconstriction in asthmatic caused by metoprolol

119. **A.** Severity of bradykinesia and akathisia caused by haloperidol
B. Severity of bradykinesia and akathisia caused by risperidone

120. **A.** Incidence of agranulocytosis caused by risperidone
B. Incidence of agranulocytosis caused by clozapine

121. **A.** Side effects in patient with liver disease taking lorazepam
B. Side effects in patient with liver disease taking diazepam

122. **A.** Magnitude of drowsiness caused by loratadine
B. Magnitude of drowsiness caused by diphenhydramine

123. **A.** In vitro anticoagulant activity of heparin
B. In vitro anticoagulant activity of Coumadin

124. **A.** Potency or efficacy of nitroglycerin as a venodilator
     B. Potency or efficacy of nitroglycerin as an arteriodilator
125. **A.** Duration of action of nitroglycerin
     B. Duration of action of isosorbide dinitrate
126. **A.** Incidence of cough in patients taking lisinopril
     B. Incidence of cough in patients taking losartan
127. **A.** Effectiveness of atenolol in treating sinus tachycardia
     B. Effectiveness of lidocaine in treating sinus tachycardia
128. **A.** Half-life of amiodarone
     B. Half-life of digoxin
129. **A.** Incidence of bone marrow suppression in patients taking vincristine
     B. Incidence of bone marrow suppression in patients taking vinblastine

CLINICAL VIGNETTES

A 56-year-old male presents to the emergency room with worsening dyspnea on exertion, orthopnea, and a 30-pound weight gain over 2 months. He has long-standing hypertension and has been taking hydrochlorothiazide. His vital signs are stable. He has jugular venous distention to 15 cm, an S3, crackles halfway up both lungs posteriorly, and 3+ pitting edema in both extremities.

130. Which initial therapeutic regimen is most appropriate?
     A. furosemide, lisinopril, carvedilol, digoxin
     B. hydrochlorothiazide, losartan, propranolol, ibuprofen
     C. dobutamine, furosemide, benazepril
     D. furosemide, captopril, digoxin
     E. amiodarone, furosemide, metoprolol
131. Assume you successfully treat this patient's condition and you see him in your office a month later for a checkup. Which of the following regimens should he be taking when he sees you in your office?
     A. furosemide, lisinopril, carvedilol, digoxin, spironolactone
     B. hydrochlorothiazide, losartan, propranolol, ibuprofen
     C. furosemide, captopril, digoxin
     D. amiodarone, furosemide, metoprolol

A 47-year-old male with a 20-year history of alcohol abuse presents to the hospital after being found down at home by a family member. The patient was lying in a pool of vomitus and was unresponsive.

REVIEW QUESTIONS

According to the paramedics, the vomitus was tinged with blood. During transport to the hospital, the patient suffered from a witnessed tonic-clonic seizure. His family members tell you he was not taking any medications, although he does have a history of bloody vomitus in the past. He has no prior history of seizures. On arrival to the emergency room, the patient is febrile to 102°F (38.8°C), has a heart rate of 130, a blood pressure of 90/30, and a respiratory rate of 33. He is disheveled and nonresponsive. He has scleral icterus, numerous spider angiomata, coarse rales at bilateral lung bases, a distended abdomen with a fluid wave, decreased bowel sounds, palmar erythema, and guaiac-positive melenic stool. You place a nasogastric tube in the emergency room and lavage out clots of bright red blood and coffee-ground material. Laboratories are as follows: WBC count 23,000 with 95% neutrophils, hemoglobin of 8.5, platelets of 100,000, BUN of 96, creatinine of 1.6, AST of 130, ALT of 90. Head CT and lumbar puncture are normal. Ascitic fluid reveals 700 WBC with 90% neutrophils, gram stain positive for gram-positive cocci in pairs. Urinalysis reveals pyuria and gram stain reveals gram-negative rods in the urine. Chest x-ray shows bilateral opacifications in the superior segments of the lower lobes.

Because you are a strong resident, you break down this complex patient into his various problems and address each individually.

132. Problem #1: infection. What is your initial antimicrobial regimen?

    A. imipenem
    B. clindamycin and oxacillin
    C. ceftriaxone
    D. erythromycin and aztreonam
    E. ceftriaxone and metronidazole

133. Problem #2: GI bleed. In addition to blood transfusion, which of the following therapeutic regimens is most appropriately initiated in the ER?

    A. DDAVP, protamine sulfate
    B. propranolol, DDAVP
    C. octreotide, DDAVP, ranitidine
    D. octreotide, ranitidine
    E. protamine sulfate, propranolol

134. Problem #3: seizure. What is your preferred antiseizure regimen?

    A. phenytoin
    B. lamotrigine
    C. phenobarbital

D. gabapentin
E. diazepam

A 66-year-old female with a history of hypertension, diabetes, and hypercholesterolemia presents to the emergency room with shortness of breath and a vague sensation of tingling in her chest. Being an astute clinician, you note her cardiac risk factors and realize that ischemia in females and diabetics is often atypical. Therefore you order an EKG as part of your evaluation. The EKG reveals 4 mm of ST elevation in leads V2 to V4. You immediately diagnose myocardial infarction (MI) and initiate the ER protocol for MI management. The patient's vital signs are: T 99.5°F (37.5°C), HR 110, BP 170/90, RR 23.

135. Which of the following adjunct therapies should be immediately offered?
    A. β-blockers, nitroglycerin, oxygen, heparin
    B. β-blockers, oxygen, ACE inhibitor, pravastatin
    C. β-blockers, oxygen, chewable aspirin, nitroglycerin
    D. calcium blockers, IV hydration, oxygen, nitroglycerin
    E. calcium blockers, oxygen, heparin, nitroglycerin

136. Which of the following are primary therapies for myocardial infarction accompanied by ST elevation?
    A. urokinase
    B. tPA plus heparin
    C. streptokinase
    D. a, b, or c

Case continued: Twenty-four hours later the patient again develops chest pain and becomes acutely short of breath. Her heart rate increases to 115, and her blood pressure falls to the 70s systolic. On exam, jugular venous distention is up from normal to 15 centimeters, there are new bibasilar rales, and an S3 is present.

137. What is the most rational pressor therapy?
    A. norepinephrine
    B. epinephrine
    C. phenylephrine and norepinephrine
    D. dopamine and dobutamine
    E. vasopressin

A 47-year-old patient with lymphoma is receiving CHOP chemotherapy (cyclophosphamide, daunorubicin, vincristine, prednisone).

138.   Which of the following are the most worrisome side effects of these four agents?
   A. alopecia, secondary leukemias, pulmonary fibrosis, Cushing's disease
   B. secondary leukemia, hemorrhagic cystitis, alopecia, hypertension
   C. hemorrhagic cystitis, cardiotoxicity, peripheral neuropathy, immunosuppression
   D. secondary leukemia, sterility, myositis, diabetes

The patient becomes neutropenic during the third cycle of CHOP therapy and presents to clinic complaining of severe abdominal pain, nausea, and vomiting. On exam, the patient's vitals are as follows: T 101°F (38.3°C), HR 130, BP 80/40, RR 34. He has marked acute distress, with peritoneal signs on abdominal exam, and hypoactive bowel sounds. WBC count is 250 cells/µL with 10% neutrophils (i.e., the patient is neutropenic). Creatinine is normal. The patient is admitted to intensive care, and surgery is called to evaluate him. You immediately begin antibiotic and pressor therapy.

139.   What antibiotic regimen is most appropriate?
   A. ampicillin, ceftazidime, metronidazole
   B. vancomycin
   C. clindamycin and azithromycin
   D. gentamicin and aztreonam
   E. ceftriaxone and erythromycin

140.   Which pressor is your agent of first choice?
   A. dobutamine
   B. digoxin
   C. epinephrine
   D. dopamine
   E. isoproterenol

A 54-year-old female with no past medical history presents to your primary care office for a routine annual exam. In the past you have twice noted that the patient had borderline elevations in blood pressure, and you have advised the rather portly woman on diet and exercise as a therapy to prevent the need for antihypertensive medications. Alas, the patient did not modify her behavior and now you again note a blood pressure of 150/90. You decide to initiate antihypertensive therapy.

141. Which therapy would you use in this patient?
     A. hydrochlorothiazide
     B. benazepril
     C. metoprolol
     D. a or b
     E. a or c

Two years later you diagnose the patient with Type II diabetes mellitus, and on screening you detect the presence of microalbuminuria.

142. What medicine would you now use to control the patient's persistent hypertension?
     A. hydrochlorothiazide
     B. benazepril
     C. metoprolol
     D. a or b
     E. a or c

ANSWERS

1. **A.** More than 50% of the drug will be protonated at a pH below 9.4 (because the pK_a represents the pH at which 50% of the drug is protonated). Therefore, in the highly acidic stomach, it will almost all be protonated, and because ionic compounds do not cross mucous membranes well, it will not be absorbed from the stomach. Because 50% of the drug is ionized at a pH of 9.4, much more than 50% will be ionized at serum pH, which is 2 logs lower (7.4). In acidic urine the drug will be ion-trapped because it will be protonated (ionized). Conversely, alkalinization of the urine will decrease the fraction of the drug that is protonated, thereby increasing reabsorption of the drug across the tubules, decreasing the drug's elimination.

2. **A.** Plasma pH is 7.4 (7.35–7.45) in normal conditions. Therefore, the drug will be at its pK_a in the plasma and, by definition, will exist as 50% ionized and 50% un-ionized. In the small intestine the drug will be deprotonated (high pH), making it negatively charged. It will therefore not be absorbed well from the small intestine. In the stomach it will be protonated, and thus electrically neutral (because it is an acid) and more easily absorbed. Alkalinizing the urine will cause more of the drug to become electrically negative, which will prevent its reabsorption across the renal tubules, increasing its excretion.

3. **C.** Partial agonists are often equally potent to full agonists, but they are less effective. That is, they bind to equal numbers of receptors at the same doses, but do not mediate a full biological effect. They also act as antagonists in the presence of a full agonist, by blocking receptors from the full agonist. Drug metabolism and pharmacokinetics (i.e., route of administration) vary from agent to agent and are in no way intrinsically related to the drug's role as an agonist, partial agonist, or antagonist.

4. **B.** Competitive antagonists reduce the binding equivalency of true agonists. That is, they decrease the potency of true agonists, mandating that higher levels of true agonist be around to achieve the same effect. However, by definition, competitive antagonism can be completely overcome by adding massive quantities of true agonists, so efficacy, or maximum biological effect, is not reduced. Conversely, irreversible antagonists remove any possibility of binding of true agonists to their receptors, in essence decreasing the maximum number of available receptors, and hence the maximal biological effect. This antagonism, by

definition, cannot be overcome by increasing the concentration of true agonist. Partial agonists often bind to receptors with equivalent affinities as do true agonists. The difference is that partial agonists are only capable of eliciting a partial biological response.

5. **E.** Drugs with high volumes of distribution move out of the vascular compartment and into tissues. They thus have lower plasma concentrations than drugs with low volumes of distribution. Volume of distribution is not related to drug metabolism or absorption in any way. Drugs with low volumes of distribution tend to be highly plasma protein bound, and vise versa, as plasma protein binding traps the drug in the vascular compartment.

6. **A.** Antiemetics are either dopamine antagonists or prokinetic 5-HT_4 agonists. Motion sickness is treated with anticholinergics such as scopolamine. Neither dopamine receptors nor 5-HT_4 receptors are involved in gastric acid production. Agonism of 5-HT_4 receptors actually stimulates gastric emptying (e.g., cisapride). The only effective therapies for gastric ulcers are acid suppression (e.g., H_2-antagonists and proton pump inhibitors) and antibiotics to eradicate *Helicobacter pylori.*

7. **E.** Clonidine activates presynaptic α_2-receptors, thereby inhibiting secretion of norepinephrine. Phentolamine and prazosin block binding of agonists to α-receptors, while tyramine and cocaine increase levels of neurotransmitters in the synaptic cleft by stimulating release from the presynaptic terminus and inhibiting reuptake by the presynaptic terminus.

8. **B.** The classic syndrome of salicylate toxicity is respiratory alkalosis, anion gap metabolic acidosis, and tinnitus. Respiratory depression is not typically seen unless coma onsets.

9. **C.** If GnRH (gonadotropin-releasing hormone) is given continuously it actually suppresses release of FSH and LH. The principal use of GnRH is to induce ovulation in women with hypothalamic amenorrhea. None of the other agents cause FSH and LH release.

10. **A.** Hydrocortisone is the synthetic equivalent to endogenous cortisone, which, by standard convention, has relative anti-inflammatory and sodium retaining potencies of 1. All other corticosteroid potencies are rated relative to hydrocortisone. Prednisolone and triamcinolone have anti-inflammatory potencies of 4 and sodium-retaining potencies of 0.25. Methylprednisolone's potencies are 5 and < 0.1, respectively, and dexamethasone and betamethasone both have anti-inflammatory

potencies of 30, with minimal sodium retention capability. Because hydrocortisone has the highest mineralocorticosteroid activity (sodium retention), it is a useful single agent for replacement of endogenous steroids in patients with adrenal failure (i.e., it replaces both corticosteroids and mineralocorticosteroids).

11. **B.** Prolonged steroid use leads to osteoporosis and can cause psychosis and femoral head necrosis. Whether or not steroids given by themselves cause ulcers remains uncertain, but in combination with other ulcer-promoting agents (e.g., NSAIDs), they increase the incidence of ulcer formation. Steroids cause hyperglycemia and can induce onset of diabetes in previously nondiabetic patients. Other prominent side effects of steroids include hypertension and immunosuppression leading to opportunistic infections.

12. **E.** First-generation sulfonylureas, and especially chlorpropamide, can cause prolonged hypoglycemia. Episodes induced by chlorpropamide can last 48 to 72 hours. Newer sulfonylureas (e.g., glyburide and glipizide) have much shorter half-lives, as do metformin and pioglitazone.

13. **C.** Metformin is a biguanide drug, whose mechanisms of action include upregulation of insulin receptors and inhibition of gluconeogenesis. Sulfonylureas (glipizide, chlorpropamide) induce insulin secretion from islet cells. Thiazolidinediones (pioglitazone) increase tissue sensitivity to insulin via genetic transcriptional changes, and acarbose inhibits α-glucosidase, which interferes with carbohydrate absorption.

14. **A-4, B-1, C-3, D-2.** The thiazolidinediones (rosiglitazone) cause peripheral volume expansion and can worsen, or cause new-onset, congestive heart failure. Acarbose causes gas and abdominal cramps. Sulfonylureas (glipizide) cause weight gain. Metformin can cause lactic acidosis in patients with renal failure. Because contrast given for CT scans or cardiac catheter can cause renal failure, the drug should be withheld the day before these procedures are performed.

15. **A & D.** Metformin does not induce insulin secretion, but instead makes insulin work more efficiently by increasing insulin receptors and also inhibiting gluconeogenesis. Thus it promotes weight loss, as opposed to sulfonylureas, which cause weight gain, and if given alone it will not cause hypoglycemia (but it can worsen hypoglycemia if given in

combination with an agent that DOES promote hypoglycemia). Metformin should be avoided in patients with renal failure and heart failure because of the risk of causing lactic acidosis.

16. **E.** Digoxin has vagomimetic activity at the AV node, thus slowing conduction through the node. For this reason it is very useful in long-term control of ventricular rate response to atrial fibrillation; it does not increase ventricular rate response to atrial fibrillation, but instead slows it down. It can also slow down sinus rhythm and can cause AV heart block and supraventricular arrhythmias. The classic digoxin-toxic patient is someone who comes in with nausea, vomiting, strange yellow-tainted vision, and a paroxysmal supraventricular tachycardia or a junctional tachycardia.

17. **C.** Cefotetan and cefoxitin are the cephalosporins (both are 2nd generation) with the highest anaerobic activity. The only other cephalosporins with acceptable activity against obligate anaerobes like *Bacteroides* spp. is ceftizoxime (3rd generation). Cefamandole is a 2nd-generation cephalosporin that is rarely used clinically because it contains a methylthiotetrazole side chain, which can inhibit vitamin K–dependent γ-carboxylation leading to a prolonged PT, and causes disulfiram-like reactions to alcohol. Cefotaxime is a 3rd-generation cephalosporin with excellent coverage of *Streptococcus pneumoniae* and community gram-negative rods, often used for meningitis, whereas cefazolin (iv) and cephalexin (po) are 1st-generation agents used for skin infections.

18. **D.** The combination of an inhibitor of dihydrofolate reductase (pyrimethamine) and a folate analog (sulfadiazine) is effective at treating *Toxoplasma*. Pentamidine is used as a 2nd-line agent against *Pneumocystis,* primaquine is used to treat the liver phase of infection in patients with *Plasmodium vivax* or *ovale*, sodium stibogluconate is used to treat leishmaniasis, and paromomycin is used to treat nematode infections.

19. **C.** Amikacin is reserved as a last-line agent because it is often active even against organisms resistant to other aminoglycosides. Tobramycin is most commonly used as an inhaled agent in patients with recurrent *Pseudomonas* infection (e.g., cystic fibrosis patients). Streptomycin is rarely used anymore because of decreased activity and increased toxicity versus other agents, whereas neomycin is given orally to wipe out colonic bacteria (since it is not absorbed) for a variety of indications, such as hepatic encephalopathy (the bacteria make nitrates absorbed by the host's gut, making the host more encephalopathic).

ANSWERS

20. **B.** Aminoglycosides are ONLY active in aerobic environments because their uptake into bacterial cells requires an oxidative process. Each of the other drugs listed has activity against anaerobes.

21. **D.** Onset of fever and fulminant diarrhea and abdominal pain after exposure to clindamycin is the CLASSIC board's question for *Clostridium difficile.* Virtually any antibiotic can lead to *C. difficile* infection, but clindamycin is a leading offender. Remember, though, that penicillins, cephalosporins, macrolides, quinolones, etc., can all cause it. Paraneoplastic syndromes can present in myriad ways, but why invoke a zebra when a very common horse is stomping outside your window? There is no evidence of acute surgical abdomen on exam, and it is hard to malinger a fever and diarrhea. Bowel metastases can cause obstruction, but should not cause prolific diarrhea.

22. **A.** The FIRST thing to do is stop the clindamycin. Even in the face of adequate therapy for *C. difficile*, if the antibiotic allowing it to colonize the gut is continued, the infection may not be eradicated. IV fluids should be given to prevent hypotension secondary to volume loss, because the diarrhea of *C. difficile* can be quite severe. Adding ampicillin and gentamicin would only worsen the problem, and stool studies will take 24 to 48 hours to come back. You can't wait that long. Enteral feeding is exactly the wrong thing to do until the colitis is resolved.

23. **D.** Metronidazole given orally is 1st-line therapy, although IV administration is usually adequate if the patient cannot tolerate POs. Clindamycin is exactly the WRONG therapy to give; it caused the problem in the first place. Ampicillin/sulbactam has very good anaerobic activity, but doesn't hit *C. difficile* well, so it will worsen the problem by wiping out additional gut flora that normally control *C. difficile* growth. Vancomycin has EXCELLENT *C. difficile* activity, equivalent to or better than metronidazole (*C. difficile* is a gram-positive rod). However, vancomycin is not secreted into the gut from the bloodstream, so IV vancomycin is useless. Oral vancomycin is a very effective alternative therapy, but because it is expensive, and more importantly, because it promotes the emergence of vancomycin-resistant *Enterococcus*, this therapy is reserved for the very rare failures of metronidazole. Giving no antibiotics is not a good option; *C. difficile* colitis can lead to acute surgical abdomen without treatment.

24. **C.** Isoniazid commonly causes B_6 deficiency, and therefore B_6 is often given in combination with isoniazid. Metabolism of the other vitamins listed is not affected.

25. **E.** Acyclovir requires herpes thymidine kinase for activity; viral resistance is linked to mutations in thymidine kinase. The other drugs require either no activation or activation by host enzymes.

26. **D.** Vinblastine causes bone marrow suppression (remember vin**b**lastine, **b**one marrow), not peripheral neuropathy. The remaining drugs all cause peripheral neuropathy.

27. **D.** Clarithromycin has no nephrotoxicity. Be aware that although vancomycin increases the risk of aminoglycoside-related nephrotoxicity, the evidence that vancomycin causes renal failure in patients with otherwise normal kidneys is scanty. Gentamicin, amphotericin B, and cisplatin are all notorious nephrotoxins.

28. **D.** Tamoxifen is an estrogen-receptor agonist/antagonist. Paclitaxel promotes microtubule assembly and inhibits disassembly, inducing apoptosis. Vincristine causes microtubule disassembly, arresting cell division in metaphase of mitosis. Colchicine prevents microtubular polymerization and function.

29. **C.** Metronidazole has the broadest obligate anaerobic bacterial spectrum available. Also, it hits protozoa, such as *Entamoeba histolytica* (amebiasis), *Trichomonas vaginalis* (trichomoniasis), and *Giardia lamblia* (giardiasis). It has no aerobic bacterial coverage.

30. **C.** Primaquine must be added to therapy for *Plasmodium vivax* or *P. ovale* to eradicate the liver phase of these organisms, or they will relapse after therapy. The remaining agents are only effective against the blood-borne parasites and do not kill latent organisms in the liver.

31. **C.** Propranolol is the first thing to do for a patient with thyroid storm. It will slow the heart rate and lower the blood pressure, thereby treating the patient hemodynamically. Furthermore, it will decrease peripheral conversion of T4 to T3, rapidly (but only slightly) reducing peripheral thyroid hormone activity. The remaining drugs act significantly more slowly, typically over days to weeks.

32. **A.** Iodinated products can inhibit release of iodinated hormone products from the thyroid. This can work in 2–3 days instead of 2–3 weeks for propylthiouracil. Propranolol does not affect thyroid hormone release from the gland. Radioactive iodine takes weeks to cause involution of the gland.

33. **A.** Ironically, although iodine-containing products can decrease release of iodinated hormone from the gland by day 2 to 3, products containing free iodine (such as sodium iodide) can also stimulate synthesis of thyroid hormone and hence can cause an initial burst of secretion of iodine hormone before inhibition kicks in. The importance of this clinically is that before administration of iodine-containing suppression therapy for thyroid storm, propylthiouracil, which inhibits iodination of thyroid hormone, must be given to the patient (see answer to question 34). Of note, organic compounds containing iodide will not induce this initial synthesis of hormone, so an iodine-containing organic molecule (such as Telepaque) is preferred to free iodine when treating thyroid storm.

34. **B.** The answer to this question follows logically from questions 32 and 33. Propylthiouracil inhibits iodination of thyroid hormone. Thus, if you want to give an iodine-containing compound to a patient in thyroid storm (which you do want to do, because, as question 32 points out, iodine is the most rapid-acting suppressor of thyroid hormone release), you must first give propylthiouracil to inhibit the tendency, pointed out in question 33, for iodine-containing products to cause an initial burst in thyroid hormone release. Thus, the order of therapy in thyroid storms is: first propranolol, second propylthiouracil, third iodine.

35. **C.** Loperamide is a narcotic derivative that binds to opioid receptors in the gut. Kaolin acts as a sort of sponge, soaking up excess fluid. The other drugs do not treat diarrhea.

36. **D.** Magnesium acts as an osmotic laxative, drawing water into the gut. The remaining drugs are not laxatives.

37. **E.** Ketamine is one of the few general anesthetic agents that does not cause cardiovascular depression. The remaining drugs can.

38. **D.** Opioids (e.g., fentanyl) plus neuroleptics induce neuroleptanalgesia.

39. **C.** Succinylcholine causes depolarization at the nerve terminus, which can lead to dangerous hyperkalemia in at-risk patients. The remaining drugs have negligible effects on potassium levels.

40. **B.** HMG-CoA reductase is the rate-limiting step in cholesterol synthesis, and inhibitors of this enzyme (the -statins) are the most effective cholesterol-reducing agents available.

41. **C.** Gemfibrozil markedly increases the risk of myositis when used in combination with HMG-CoA reductase inhibitors.

42. **E.** Niacin is the most effective reducer of serum triglyceride levels.

43. **A.** Cholestyramine causes loss of bile salts in the GI tract, stimulating the enzyme 7-hydroxylase to break down cholesterol in order to synthesize more bile salts.

44. **B.** MAO inhibitors can induce hypertensive crisis when large amounts of tyramine-containing foods are ingested.

45. **D.** Dopamine receptor agonists block prolactin secretion, and thus are useful in treating prolactinomas.

46. **C.** Chronic use of L-dopa/carbidopa can induce hyperkinesia/ dyskinesias, including facial grimacing, rhythmic jerking movements of hands, head-bobbing, chewing, and lip-smacking (tardive dyskinesias).

47. **A.** Phencyclidine induces psychotic episodes.

48. **D.** Patients often see sounds, hear colors, smell sights, etc., while taking LSD.

49. **E.** On any exam, any time you are asked about pinpoint pupils, you should always think immediately of opioids.

50. **B.** Metoclopramide and droperidol are commonly used antiemetics that work by blocking D_2 receptors in the emetic center of the CNS.

51. **A.** Ondansetron and granisetron both antagonize 5-HT$_3$ receptors in the emetic center of the CNS.

52. **E.** Buspirone is an anxiolytic that works by agonizing central 5-HT$_1$ receptors.

53. **A.** The cholinergic system bronchoconstricts, and the adrenergic system bronchodilates. Blocking cholinergic signaling to the bronchioles therefore causes bronchodilation.

54. **C.** Corticosteroids, preferably inhaled because of diminished toxicity, are always given to severe asthmatics with frequent attacks in order to effect a prolonged decrease in airway inflammation. Cromolyn is not effective enough for severe asthmatics and is only used to prevent attacks in mild but chronic asthmatics.

55. **B.** No drug is more effective for acute symptomatic relief than albuterol. Although it very effectively bronchodilates asthmatics, it does not prevent airway inflammation, and thus can only be used for short-term symptom relief, not long-term prevention of attacks.

56. **E.** Theophylline is rarely used nowadays because of its very narrow therapeutic window and severe toxicity (seizures).

57. **D.** Cromolyn stabilizes mast cell membranes, preventing degranulation that sets off an asthmatic attack.

58. **B.** According to national guidelines (Joint National Committee on Hypertension), thiazide diuretics and β-blockers are the only two 1st-line agents for isolated essential hypertension (not accompanied by other comorbidities).

59. **C.** Spironolactone reduces all-cause mortality in patients with severe heart failure. No other diuretic has been proven to do this in a prospective randomized study.

60. **D.** Acetazolamide inhibits carbonic anhydrase in the renal tubule, causing bicarbonate wasting in the urine. This leads to a hyperchloremic nongap metabolic acidosis.

61. **A.** Because it is so effective a diuretic, most heart failure patients are put on furosemide to maintain water balance.

62. **A-1 or 3; B-2; C-1, 2, 6; D-4; E-3; F-2; G-1, 2, 5.** β-blockers and thiazide diuretics are the only two 1st-line drugs for essential hypertension. ACE inhibitors decrease the risk of renal failure, mortality, strokes, and myocardial infarctions in diabetics or those with severe peripheral vascular disease. β-blockers, ACE inhibitors, and HMG-CoA reductase inhibitors reduce long-term mortality in patients who have survived a myocardial infarction. α_1-antagonists can simultaneously treat hypertension and BPH and are therefore 1st-line antihypertensives in patients with benign prostatic hypertrophy (BPH). Because thiazides decrease calcium excretion in the urine, they are 1st-line antihypertensive agents for patients with osteoporosis. ACE inhibitors decrease proteinuria regardless of the cause of proteinuria. β-blockers, ACE inhibitors, and spironolactone have each been proven to decrease mortality in patients with congestive heart failure.

63. **A.** Melphalan is an alkylating agent, meaning that it causes DNA cross-linking. All alkylating agents cause bone marrow suppression and alopecia. Melphalan does not cause significant renal or bladder toxicity.

64. **B.** Bleomycin causes pulmonary fibrosis, as does the other "killer B" drug, busulfan.

65. **C.** Cisplatin's predominant toxicity is vomiting and renal failure, with minimal bone marrow suppression, in contrast to carboplatin. Cisplatin also causes ototoxicity and peripheral neuropathy.

66. **D.** Doxorubicin, and all anthracyclines, cause cardiac toxicity, leading to a dose-dependent dilated cardiomyopathy.

67. **F.** Imatinib mesylate (Gleevec) is a new drug for the therapy of chronic myeloid leukemia (CML). CML is caused by the *bcr:abl* translocation, which creates a tyrosine kinase enzyme lacking its normal inhibitory domain. This leads to uninhibited tyrosine kinase activity, which translates into uninhibited cell proliferation. Imatinib mesylate was targeted/designed to inhibit the defective tyrosine kinase molecule. It is thus one of the first targeted/ designed agents available for use (protease inhibitors for AIDS were also targeted/designed) and is spurring hopes that the huge investment we've made in basic science will soon, finally, pay off with new therapies for cancer.

68. **A.** Leucovorin is folinic acid, the product of dihydrofolate reductase. Thus, it bypasses the inhibition in the enzyme caused by methotrexate, rescuing patients from the drug's toxicity.

69. **C.** Allopurinol inhibits xanthine oxidase, which breaks down metabolites in the purine pathway. Allopurinol thus inhibits degradation of 6-mercaptopurine, thereby increasing its activity and toxicity. Conversely, azathioprine requires xanthine oxidase for conversion to the active drug, 6-mercaptopurine, thus allopurinol inhibits the activity of azathioprine.

70. **E.** Carmustine penetrates the CNS well, whereas most chemotherapy agents do not.

71. **C.** Trimethoprim inhibits dihydrofolate reductase.

72. **E.** Oxacillin is a member of the penicillinase-resistant penicillin class. Resistance of *Staphylococcus aureus* to penicillins is principally caused by secretion of β-lactamase, and drugs like oxacillin are resistant to the β-lactamases. Methicillin-resistant *S. aureus* (MRSA, which is the same as oxacillin-resistant *S. aureus*) has a different mechanism of resistance: altered penicillin-binding proteins.

ANSWERS

73. **A.** Sulfasalazine is not absorbed from the GI tract. It is degraded in the GI tract by bacteria secreting lytic enzymes, releasing the two components sulfapyridine and 5-aminosalicylate. 5-aminosalicylate is the active component, working as a local anti-inflammatory agent in inflammatory bowel disease. Sulfapyridine is a carrier molecule.

74. **B.** Ceftazidime is a 3rd-generation cephalosporin with extended gram-negative activity. It is commonly used to treat *Pseudomonas*, or other nasty nosocomial gram-negative infections. The other antimicrobials listed have poor or no gram-negative coverage.

75. **D.** Amoxicillin has very good oral bioavailability. Trimethoprim has acceptable oral bioavailability, but less than amoxicillin; the remaining drugs are given parenterally.

76. **E.** Ceftriaxone and cefotaxime (3rd-generation cephalosporins) have very good CNS penetration and cover the major meningitis pathogens, including *Streptococcus pneumoniae*, *Neisseria meningitidis,* and *Haemophilus influenzae.* Aztreonam penetrates the CNS well (as do all β-lactams), but it only covers gram-negative agents. Levofloxacin also has excellent *S. pneumoniae* coverage, but there are minimal outcomes data with it in meningitis, so its use is not recommended.

77. **C.** Cilastatin inhibits the degradation of imipenem in renal tubular brush border cells. Without adding cilastatin, imipenem would have a very short half-life.

78. **B.** Aztreonam is a β-lactam derivative that is much less susceptible to β-lactamase production by bacteria. Although it has excellent, highly broad-spectrum gram-negative activity, even against nosocomial pathogens, it has no activity against anaerobes or gram-positive organisms

79. **A.** Because of its size, vancomycin is not absorbed at all when given orally. This makes it ideal therapy for resistant *C. difficile*, because extremely high levels of vancomycin are achievable in stool because it is not absorbed.

80. **D.** Dosing fluoroquinolones orally is essentially identical to dosing them IV if the gut is working (e.g., not edematous, not obstructed). The only reason ever to dose a fluoroquinolone intravenously is if the patient is not tolerating POs.

81. **C.** Gray-baby syndrome is a devastating, highly lethal potential side effect of chloramphenicol, caused by poisoning of mitochondria in the infant.

82. **D.** In general, doxycycline is a very benign agent, but one side effect that is relatively common to all tetracyclines is the development of sunburn (can be severe) when people taking the drug are exposed to a lot of sun. Patients should use sunblock while taking doxycycline.

83. **E.** Aminoglycosides do not penetrate gram-positive organisms well because of the size of the antibiotics and the thick peptidoglycan wall that protects gram-positive bacteria. However, addition of a cell-wall inhibitor, classically a β-lactam agent, opens pores in the cell wall, which improves aminoglycoside penetration. Once the aminoglycoside is inside the bacteria, it inhibits protein synthesis, preventing repair of the already damaged cell wall. The result is synergistic killing between aminoglycosides and cell-wall active agents.

84. **B.** Rifampin is extremely broad spectrum, covering gram-positive cocci and rods, gram-negative cocci and rods, anaerobes, and many atypical organisms. However, resistance commonly develops to rifampin when it is used as monotherapy, so it is almost always combined with a second agent in clinical practice.

85. **A.** Oral erythromycin can cause prominent nausea, vomiting, and dyspepsia, which can make it difficult to tolerate.

86. **C.** Another highly lethal, if rare (1 in 50,000 pts), side effect of chloramphenicol is idiosyncratic, often irreversible aplastic anemia.

87. **D.** Isoniazid is one of the classic causes of drug-induced lupus.

88. **A.** Patients on prolonged ethambutol need to have regular vision checks to identify this toxicity early.

89. **B.** Rifampin typically causes urine, saliva, and tears to turn bright orange.

90. **E.** Vancomycin is the cause of the favorite board's topic, "red man syndrome." This is an allergic reaction causing rash, facial flushing, and sometimes airway obstruction. The general consensus is that it is not an allergy to vancomycin itself, but to some contaminant in the preparation. Over the last several

decades, this syndrome has become increasingly rare in clinical practice, as purification of the drug has improved.

91. **E.** Patients taking indinavir need to drink large amounts of water to prevent this side effect.

92. **D.** Lamivudine is a 1st-line therapy for both HIV and hepatitis B virus (hepatitis B has a reverse transcriptase as part of its life cycle).

93. **C.** Stavudine acts via a similar mechanism of AZT, and the two drugs are not combined because they are felt to be antagonistic (definitely seen in the test tube, probably seen in early clinical trials).

94. **A.** Initially there was excitement about using nevirapine as a postexposure prophylaxis following needlesticks, but several people have died from fulminant hepatitis caused by the drug.

95. **B.** Competing nucleoside synthesis is inhibited by hydroxyurea (inhibits ribonucleotide reductase), thereby increasing the relative drug level of didanosine inside the cell.

96. **A-7, B-11, C-8, D-10, E-1, F-13, G-15, H-5, I-6, J-3, K-12, L-9, M-4, N-2, O-14.**

97. **B, C, F** are all monoclonal antibodies.

98. **G.** G-CSF is granulocyte-colony stimulating factor, a recombinant cytokine that stimulates marrow production of neutrophils.

99. **E.** Imatinib mesylate inhibits the tyrosine kinase that causes CML cells to replicate uncontrollably.

100. **A.** All-trans-retinoic-acid (ATRA) induces the differentiation of cells in a subtype of AML (M3 AML = promyelocytic leukemia). The cells have a specific translocation that affects the retinoic acid receptor. ATRA is thus useful as induction chemotherapy, but still must be followed by standard chemotherapy for consolidation.

101. **A, B, C, D, E**

102. **F.** Naloxone is a short-acting opiate antagonist. It used to diagnose opiate overdose by assessing for very rapid reversal of coma, pinpoint pupils, and respiratory depression. It must be repeatedly dosed every few hours to truly treat an opiate overdose.

103. **H.** Diphenhydramine has anticholinergic properties that make it an ideal antidote for acute dystonic reactions to dopamine antagonists (restores the normal dopamine/cholinergic signal balance).

104. **G.** Dimercaprol is a heavy-metal chelator.

105. **C.** Pralidoxime regenerates acetylcholinesterase by breaking the irreversible bond between it and the organophosphate. If the bond "ages" pralidoxime is not effective, so it must be given as soon as possible after the overdose.

106. **B.** Digibind binds to digoxin in the bloodstream and limits its activity.

107. **A.** If given in time, *N*-acetylcysteine completely prevents toxicity from acetaminophen. It is a true antidote.

108. **D.** Mesna absorbs the toxic metabolite of ifosfamide or high-dose cyclophosphamide that causes hemorrhagic cystitis.

109. **E.** Nitrites (amyl or sodium) induce formation of methemoglobin in the blood. As methemoglobin has higher affinity for cyanide than mitochondrial cytochrome oxidase, this frees the oxidative phosphorylation cascade of cyanide by causing the cyanide to bind to methemoglobin. Nitrite administration is followed by sodium thiosulfate administration, which converts cyanide bound to the methemoglobin to thiocyanate, which can be urinated out.

110. **D.** Dopamine is almost always the first pressor given to a run-of-the-mill hypotensive patient. It acts by both β_1- and α_1-receptors, thereby increasing heart rate, contractility, and peripheral vascular resistance. At low doses it binds to dopamine receptors that cause renal vasodilation, and it promotes diuresis.

111. **B.** Norepinephrine is an extremely potent vasoconstrictor, acting by binding to α_1-receptors, and is therefore most useful in cases with low systemic vascular resistance. However, it can lead to profound tachycardia because of very potent β_1 activity, and this can be undesirable if a patient is ischemic or is already markedly tachycardic. Prolonged use may lead to limb ischemia.

112. **C.** Phenylephrine is a strict α_1 agonist, with no β agonist effects. It is a potent vasoconstrictor, like norepinephrine, and is therefore most useful in patients with low systemic vascular resistance. Its advantage over norepinephrine is that, because it has no β-agonist effects, it does NOT promote tachycardia and may even cause autonomic reflex bradycardia if a patient who is baseline tachycardic and hypotensive approaches normal blood pressure on the drug. Many people prefer this agent to norepinephrine in markedly tachycardic or ischemic patients for this reason. However, phenylephrine may also cause coronary

vasoconstriction, so in ischemic, hypotensive patients, you may be damned if you do and damned if you don't.

113. **E.** Because dobutamine is an almost pure β_1 agonist, it is the preferred agent for patients in cardiogenic shock. It dramatically improves cardiac contractility and cardiac output, which can elevate blood pressure if the hypotension is due to low output and can also decrease wedge pressure, thereby effectively treating pulmonary edema. However, because it has no vasoconstrictive properties, the increased cardiac output may lead to autonomic reflex vasodilation, which can potentially drop blood pressure even more. Therefore, in hypotensive patients, it is prudent to combine dobutamine with dopamine.

114. **A.** This is an easy one. If someone is without a pulse, you give epinephrine. Period. First you start your ABCs (airway, breathing, cardiac). Get a rhythm monitor on the patient, and if they are in ventricular fibrillation or tachycardia, you shock them. Otherwise give them epinephrine IV and begin chest compressions and ventilatory support (bag mask or intubate). Every cause of pulselessness is treated with epinephrine, including V-fib/V-tach, pulseless electrical activity, and asystole (whereas vasopressin is used only in pulselessness secondary to V-fib/V-tach; see question 116). Epinephrine can be given as a drip to be used as a pressor, but this is not very commonly done.

115. **G.** Digoxin is useful as a pressor because it improves cardiac contractility without increasing heart rate or afterload and with only a minimal increase in myocardial oxygen demand.

116. **F.** On the basis of animal data, several nonrandomized studies, and one small randomized study in Europe, vasopressin is now included as 1st-line therapy for pulseless ventricular fibrillation or tachycardia in the 2000 ACLS guidelines. It can be given as a one-time dose in lieu of the initial epinephrine dose for this condition. It should be given AFTER electrical cardioversion is attempted three times, or right away if cardioversion is not immediately available. It is NOT recommended to repeat the dose. If the patient continues to be pulseless, epinephrine can be given as normal during the code. Vasopressin can also be given as a drip pressor for hypotension.

117. **B.** Pilocarpine has better CNS and ocular penetration because it is nonionized and nonpolar.

118. **A.** Bronchoconstriction is caused by β_2-blockade. Propranolol is a nonselective β-blocker, whereas metoprolol preferentially

blocks β_1 over β_2, as does atenolol. Betaxolol is even more selective toward β_1. Hence propranolol has the most β_2 blockade, and thus has the greatest potential to cause bronchoconstriction.

119. **A.** High-potency typical antipsychotics, otherwise known as neuroleptics, are potent blockers of D_2 receptors and caused marked movement disorders. Lower-potency neuroleptics cause somewhat fewer movement disorders but more anticholinergic side effects. Atypical antipsychotics have markedly diminished propensity to induce movement disorders. Risperidone is such a drug, although even newer atypicals, such as olanzapine and quetiapine, cause still less movement disorders. Clozapine causes essentially none. Haloperidol is a classic high-potency agent, carrying a significant risk of inducing movement disorders with prolonged use.

120. **B.** Although clozapine causes even fewer movement disorders than risperidone, clozapine causes agranulocytosis in 1–5% of people taking it. Risperidone does not cause agranulocytosis.

121. **B.** Lorazepam is not metabolized in the liver, unlike diazepam, so it is safer to use in patients with liver disease.

122. **B.** Older antihistamines cause marked drowsiness. Newer agents have less anticholinergic activity and hence less drowsiness.

123. **A.** Heparin speeds up anticoagulation mediated by antithrombin III, which is present in the test tube. Coumadin acts as an enzyme inhibitor in the liver. It is only active in vivo and has no effects in a test tube.

124. **A.** Nitroglycerin is far more active on veins than arteries. It thus lowers preload much more than afterload, in addition to causing coronary vasodilation.

125. **B.** Isosorbide dinitrate has a much longer circulating half-life than nitroglycerin, slowly releasing nitric oxide as it circulates.

126. **A.** One of the most common side effects in patients taking ACE inhibitors is nagging cough, caused by the inhibition of the breakdown of bradykinin. ACE receptor blockers do not cause this side effect, as they do not inhibit bradykinin breakdown.

127. **A.** β-blockers slow the heart rate. Lidocaine has no effect on normally depolarized tissue. It only works to convert ventricular tachycardia or fibrillation.

128. **A.** Amiodarone has a half-life of up to 3 months; digoxin is on the order of 24 hours.

129. **B.** This is a key differentiating factor between these otherwise similar drugs. Remember, vinblastine causes bone marrow suppression, whereas vincristine causes peripheral neuropathy.

130. **D.** The primary therapy for patients in acute congestive heart failure (CHF) is rapid and aggressive diuresis. The diuretic should be given intravenously because bowel-wall edema can prevent absorption of medications across the gastrointestinal tract. Intravenous furosemide is the preferred diuretic therapy. You would NOT give hydrochlorothiazide because it has weaker intrinsic diuretic activity than furosemide, cannot be dosed intravenously, and the patient has already failed thiazide therapy. Although any ACE inhibitor can and should be used in patients in CHF (unless renal failure accompanies it), captopril is the preferred initial agent for acutely ill patients because it can be dosed three times per day and therefore can most rapidly be titrated up to a therapeutic dose. Digoxin should definitely be used in an acute setting as a positive inotrope that minimally increases myocardial oxygen demand. β-blockers are CONTRAINDICATED in patients in ACUTE CHF. This patient has obvious fluid overload, with rales on exam. β-blockers should be initiated once the patient's fluid status has normalized, typically as an outpatient once other therapies are at stable doses. The only β-blockers studied in CHF are bisoprolol (mixed results), metoprolol, and carvedilol, the latter two of which have been beneficial in all studies and are therefore preferred. There is no indication for antiarrhythmic agents other than β-blockers in CHF (unless the patient has had a cardiac arrest due to ventricular arrhythmia, in which case amiodarone can be used). NSAIDs should be assiduously avoided (except for aspirin) because they can worsen tenuous glomerular filtration in CHF patients, leading to worsening fluid retention and hence worsening CHF. Because this patient has normal vital signs, there is no indication for pressors, such as dobutamine.

131. **A.** Although thiazides can be used to maintain fluid status in patients with mild CHF, typically loop diuretics are preferred because of their greater intrinsic activity. ACE inhibitors should be given to every CHF patient if they are tolerated, and although captopril is preferred for rapid titration in hospital, other ACE inhibitors are preferred for outpatient therapy because they can be dosed once or twice a day instead of three times per day. β-blockers, specifically carvedilol or metoprolol, are now considered standard-of-care for CHF patients who are diuresed to dry weight and are on a stable medical regimen

(e.g., not acutely in failure). Spironolactone reduces mortality in patients with CHF and is now standard-of-care. Digoxin does not improve mortality, but it does improve exercise tolerance and reduce hospitalization; it should be used if tolerated, but is clearly less important than other therapies that reduce mortality.

132. **E.** Breaking down this patient by problem list is exactly what you need to do. The problems are too many and too complex to deal with en masse. Starting with the infectious issue, the first thing to do when deciding which antibiotics to use is to decide what infections are present, what organisms are likely to cause those infections, and what the expected resistance patterns might be. This patient clearly has a pneumonia, and given that he was found unconscious in a pool of vomitus, lying on his back, and the pneumonia is in both lungs at the superior segments of the lower lobes, this is almost certainly an aspiration pneumonia. Therefore, anaerobic coverage is going to be crucial to cover bowel flora. He also has spontaneous bacterial peritonitis (ascitic fluid neutrophils > 250/mL, and gram stain positive) with what is certainly going to be *Streptococcus pneumoniae* (gram-positive cocci in pairs in ascitic fluid; *S. pneumoniae* is a common cause of spontaneous bacterial peritonitis). Finally, he has a gram-negative rod urinary tract infection. Thus three types of organisms need to be covered: anaerobes, *Strep*, and gram-negative rods. Yes, imipenem covers all these, but it also lowers seizure threshold and can precipitate seizures. Furthermore, broad-spectrum agents like imipenem should be used as agents of last choice to prevent the spread of bacterial resistance. Clindamycin is adequate for the anaerobic aspiration pneumonia and has reasonable *Strep* coverage, but it does not cover gram negatives at all, nor does oxacillin. Ceftriaxone is excellent therapy for both *Strep* and gram-negative rods, but lacks anaerobic activity. Aztreonam covers gram negatives exclusively, and erythromycin has some *Strep* coverage; neither cover anaerobes well. Thus, the best combination offered is ceftriaxone and metronidazole, the former for gram-negative rods and *Strep*, and the latter for bowel anaerobes.

133. **D.** Given this patient's alcohol history and clear signs of cirrhosis on exam, acute variceal bleeding from portal hypertension must be high on the differential diagnosis of this patient's upper-GI bleed. Hence, octreotide should be initiated as soon as possible, because it is proven to decrease the incidence of variceal rebleeding. Ranitidine given intravenously should also be initiated, because gastric ulcer and gastritis are also potential causes of bleeding (increasingly, clinicians are using proton pump

inhibitors in lieu of H_2-blockers in this setting). Ideally, endoscopy should be performed to discern the etiology of the bleed and offer therapeutic intervention. Propranolol is an effective therapy for prevention of variceal bleeding by reducing portal pressures; however, in an acute bleed with a low blood pressure, it should be held. Once the bleed is finished and the patient is hemodynamically stable, propranolol should be started before discharge to reduce the risk of rebleeding. DDAVP is useful in the treatment of bleeding disorders caused by platelet dysfunction (e.g., some forms of von Willebrand's disease and renal failure). Protamine sulfate is used as a heparin antidote. The latter two agents have no role in this patient.

134. **E.** This patient almost certainly had an alcohol withdrawal seizure. Benzodiazepines are the preferred therapy for these types of seizures, as well as for alcohol withdrawal in general. The other medications will be much less efficacious. Especially considering this patient's underlying liver disease, phenytoin should probably be avoided.

135. **C.** This is an easy one. If you EVER get ANY questions on the boards about therapy for chest pain, ischemia, or infarction, the right answer will ALWAYS have aspirin in it. Everyone gets an aspirin unless they are actively massively bleeding right in front of your eyes (even guaiac-positive patients or those with minor active bleeding should still get the aspirin!). Chewable is preferred because it is absorbed more rapidly, but this is a minor point. The major point is: never forget the aspirin! In addition, β-blockade in ischemic patients is a cornerstone of therapy, reducing myocardial oxygen demand and thereby minimizing the gap between oxygen demand and supply. Oxygen and nitroglycerin should also be given. The role of heparin in transmural myocardial infarction is open to question. Although heparin is of proven benefit in unstable angina and so-called non–ST-elevation myocardial infarction, in large randomized studies it has not been shown to be of significant benefit in patients with transmural, ST-elevation myocardial infarctions unless it is used in conjunction with tPA. In the latter instance, the use of heparin is not as primary therapy for the infarct, but rather to prevent the transient thrombogenic potential caused by tPA.

136. **D.** Streptokinase and urokinase are acceptable alternatives to tPA, although most clinicians prefer tPA. In large randomized

studies, tPA does appear to have a small benefit over the other two drugs, although the number of patients needed to treat to demonstrate this benefit is very large.

137. **D.** The pressor that is most desirable in this setting is clearly dobutamine. This patient appears to be suffering from acute cardiogenic shock (i.e., pump failure). That is, the shock is not due to peripheral vasodilation or loss of circulating volume, but to failure of the heart to pump that volume forward. Unfortunately, dobutamine may cause a mild decrease in blood pressure and often must be given in conjunction with dopamine to prevent this decrease.

138. **C.** Although cyclophosphamide can cause alopecia and secondary leukemias, its most famous and specific adverse effect is hemorrhagic cystitis. The classic and most concerning toxicity seen with daunorubicin is cardiotoxicity, which is dose-dependent. Vincristine causes peripheral neuropathy. Steroids can induce diabetes or hypertension, but the most concerning side effect is inhibition of cell-mediated immunity.

139. **A.** According to Infectious Disease Society of America guidelines, empiric antibiotic regimens in neutropenic patients without a clear source of infection require inclusion of an agent that covers nosocomial gram-negative rods because these infections are common and highly lethal in neutropenic patients. Gram-positive coverage is optional, as is double gram-negative coverage for *Pseudomonas*. However, this patient has an obvious source on exam: the abdomen. The ceftazidime has excellent, broad-spectrum gram-negative coverage, including nosocomial gram-negative rods. The metronidazole is the broadest spectrum anaerobic agent available, and because gut flora is 99% anaerobic, clearly such coverage is mandatory in a patient with an acute abdomen. The ampicillin covers *Enterococcus*, which is a fastidious facultative anaerobe often found in the gut. Vancomycin alone is clearly inadequate, as it offers no gram-negative or anaerobic coverage. Clindamycin might replace metronidazole for anaerobic coverage, although clindamycin has poorer activity against *Bacteroides* spp., the most common organisms in the bowel, but azithromycin offers totally inadequate gram-negative coverage. Gentamicin and aztreonam would be adequate coverage for a neutropenic patient with no clear source, double-covering for nosocomial gram-negative rods, but neither drug covers anaerobes or gram positives at all. Finally, ceftriaxone

does have broad-spectrum gram-negative coverage, but it does not cover nosocomial gram negatives as well as ceftazidime or aminoglycosides, and neither it nor erythromycin has much anaerobic coverage.

140. **D.** Dopamine is the 1st-line agent here, because the main thing needed in this patient is an increase in systemic vascular resistance. Phenylephrine and norepinephrine would also be acceptable alternatives, although most clinicians start with dopamine unless there are reasons to avoid worsening tachycardia, in which case phenylephrine is more useful. The major effect of dobutamine, digoxin, epinephrine, and isoproterenol is to increase cardiac output rather than vascular resistance, so these agents would not be 1st line in this patient.

141. **E.** According to consensus national guidelines, initial therapy for hypertension in a patient with no other comorbid illnesses should include either a thiazide diuretic or a β-blocker. This is because only agents from these two classes have been shown to improve mortality in this patient population. ACE inhibitors have not been studied in this patient population. For the time being, they are not on the recommended list for initial therapy of isolated hypertension.

142. **B.** The patient now clearly has a 1st-line indication for ACE inhibitor therapy. ACE inhibitors are 1st-line antihypertensive agents in patients with diabetes and proteinuria (and many clinicians feel they are 1st line in all diabetics, whether or not they have proteinuria), peripheral vascular disease, and a history of myocardial infarction or low ejection fractions.

INDEX